The Recovery *Workbook*

▼▼▼

Practical Coping and Empowerment Strategies for People with Psychiatric Disability

LeRoy Spaniol
Martin Koehler
Dori Hutchinson

CENTER FOR PSYCHIATRIC REHABILITATION

Sargent College of Health and Rehabilitation Sciences
Boston University

Published by:
Center for Psychiatric Rehabilitation
Sargent College of Health and Rehabilitation Sciences
Boston University
940 Commonwealth Avenue West
Boston, MA 02215

This publication was supported in part by a grant from the National Institute on Disability and Rehabilitation Research and the Center for Mental Health Services.

Printed in the United States of America

ISBN 13: 978-1-878512-01-7
ISBN10: 1-878512-01-3

Center for Psychiatric Rehabilitation
Sargent College of Health and Rehabilitation Sciences
Boston University

The Recovery Workbook

▼▼▼

Practical Coping and Empowerment Strategies for People with Psychiatric Disability

Chapter One:
Introduction
1 Purpose of the Workbook
3 Goals of the Workbook
3 Suggestions for Getting Started

Chapter Two:
Recovery
11 The Process of Recovery
12 Phases of the Recovery Process
15 Aspects of the Recovery Process

Chapter Three:
Increasing Knowledge and Control
23 The Impact of Serious Mental Illness
26 The Services of a Recovery-Oriented Mental Health System
28 The Values of a Recovery-Oriented Mental Health System

Chapter Four:
Managing Life's Stresses
33 Symptoms of Stress
43 Sources of Stress
49 Coping Strategies

Chapter Five:
Enhancing Personal Meaning
71 Acknowledging Our Accomplishments
74 Personal Enrichment

Chapter Six:
Building Personal Support
83 Connecting
84 Basic Communication Skills
92 Asking for Support
95 Setting Boundaries on Our Relationships

Chapter Seven:
Setting Personal Goals
99 A Step-By-Step Guide for Setting Personal Goals
105 Developing a Plan for Achieving a Personal Goal

113 Bibliography

The Authors   **LeRoy Spaniol, PhD,** is a licensed psychologist who has extensive experience leading workshops in divorce adjustment, stress management, writing skills, self-esteem, assertiveness skills, and other issues. He is research associate professor in the Department of Rehabilitation Counseling at Boston University, adjunct associate professor of counseling psychology at Boston University, executive publisher of the *Psychiatric Rehabilitation Journal*, and associate executive director of the Center for Psychiatric Rehabilitation, Boston University.

Martin Koehler, BA, is a research assistant at the Center for Psychiatric Rehabilitation and a graduate of Harvard College. He has also completed a certificate in public interest law at the College of Public and Community Service at the University of Massachusetts. He is active in mental health politics in Massachusetts.

Dori Hutchinson, MS, ScD, is coordinator of instructional services in the Career Services Division at the Center for Psychiatric Rehabilitation, Boston University. She is an instructor in the Department of Rehabilitation Counseling at Boston University teaching courses in case management, clinical skills, and direct skills teaching. She has done extensive research in fitness and mental illness. Ms. Hutchinson is also involved in a community service project, working with high-risk students in the Boston public school system to increase their sense of self-determination, empowerment, and choice.

No royalties are paid to the authors of this book. All proceeds from the sale of this book are used to further the work of the Center for Psychiatric Rehabilitation.

Acknowledgments   We thank the many people with whom we piloted this workbook. They shared their experiences willingly and generously, knowing that others might benefit from what they have learned.

We also give special thanks to Mikal Cohen and William Anthony for their many useful suggestions on the text and the exercises.

CHAPTER 1 *Introduction*

Purpose of the Workbook

Recovery is a common human experience. We all experience recovery at some point in our lives from injury, from illness, or from trauma. Psychiatric disability has a devastating impact on the lives of people who experience it. It is devastating because people with psychiatric disability are left profoundly disconnected from themselves, from others, from their environments, and from meaning or purpose in life. While the illness itself causes people to feel disconnected, stigma (negative personal, professional, and societal values, attitudes, and practices) further disconnects people and represents a serious barrier to building new connections.

Recovery is the process by which people with psychiatric disability rebuild and further develop these important personal, social, environmental, and spiritual connections, and confront the devastating effects of stigma through personal empowerment. Recovery is a process of adjusting one's attitudes, feelings, perceptions, beliefs, roles, and goals in life. It is a process of self-discovery, self-renewal, and transformation. Recovery is a deeply emotional process. Recovery involves creating a new personal vision for oneself. Recovering from the illness and from stigma can be very stressful. We have written this workbook as a resource for people with psychiatric disability, to help them in their recovery process and to help them to prevent, eliminate, or cope with the stressors in their lives. We believe that it is never too late to begin the recovery process. Understanding the recovery process and our own recovery experience are important first steps in returning to a life that is fulfilling for ourselves and contributing to others.

The coping and empowerment strategies presented in this workbook relate to this process we call "recovery." Recovery is not a concept that is commonly applied to understanding the impact of severe mental illness. It has had far greater acceptance in the field of physical illness. People with physical disability have long advocated to be seen as people first—people who happen to have a disability. While a serious physical disability such as paraplegia may result in a person being confined to a wheelchair for the remainder of his/her life—the person can change dramatically over the course of time. He/she can come to terms with the disability and its chronicity and still have a life for him/herself. This is called recovery. The disability does not go away but the person recovers. For people with psychiatric disability, the focus has typically been more on the illness than on the person with the illness. The focus has been on symptoms rather than on how to increase functioning. People with psychiatric disability have rarely been taught about the possibility of recovery. Unfortunately, neither have professionals or family members been taught about recovery. The acknowledgment of the recovery process, and the contribution a person can make toward his/her own recovery, has only recently been recognized. The recovery process is described in Chapter Two.

Tensions within the mental health system and among those who collaborate with people with psychiatric disability in their recovery process (i.e., the family, other people with psychiatric disability, professionals, etc.) result from a lack of clarity of and support for the process of recovery, the means to make it more effective, and the roles that each one plays in this process. Tensions are further increased by the profound feelings and emotions aroused by this lack of clarity and support.

Diversity within the mental health system and among those who collaborate with people with psychiatric disability in their recovery process results from the strengths and limitations each individual brings to the process of clarifying and supporting the process of recovery, the means to make it more effective, and the roles that each one plays in this process. Diversity can be a source of tension or it can be a source of enormous creativity if it is acknowledged and respected.

Collaboration can be built within the mental health system and among those who assist people with psychiatric disability in their recovery process by actively working together to clarify and support the process of recovery, the means to make it more effective, and the roles that each person plays in this process. A commitment to working through the tensions resulting from lack of clarity and support, and a commitment to respecting the diversity of strengths and limitations people bring to this process, will enhance collaboration and the building of new connections for people with psychiatric disability.

This workbook offers the potential of building our life again—of picking up the threads of personal, social, and vocational growth that were so profoundly interrupted by the psychiatric disability. The authors hope that this workbook will provide the information and the skills needed to strengthen the recovery process, to cope more creatively, and to live life more fully.

Goals of the Workbook

The specific goals of the workbook are:

1. To become aware of the recovery process.
2. To increase knowledge and control.
3. To become aware of the importance and nature of stress.
4. To enhance personal meaning.
5. To build personal support.
6. To develop goals and a plan of action.

The material has been developed to allow the workbook to be used as part of a training workshop, course, or seminar conducted by a consumer leader(s); or to be used by individuals for their own self-study.

Suggestions for Getting Started

Step 1: Make a decision to start changing your life and to assume responsibility for your recovery process. Decide that you are worth it. Give yourself a generous amount of time to change—and then add some more time. We tend to change in stages or percentages rather than all at once. And we frequently find ourselves continuing behaviors we are trying to change. Simply acknowledge that you still have a way to go and do not be critical of yourself. Change, even when we want it, takes time and patience.

Step 2: Make a commitment to action; to taking the necessary steps to bring about the changes you want, e.g., decide now that you will complete the whole workbook.

Step 3: Build some immediate satisfiers into your life. Plan to do something that takes care of you *every day*, e.g. taking a walk, listening to music, spending time with a friend. This will begin to break the cycle of stress in your life. Build some special satisfiers into your life on a weekly basis, e.g., a trip to the library or to the beach. Focusing on enriching your life while you deal with recovery issues will help you to move your new energy into positive directions for yourself.

Step 4: Start with someone. Choose someone with whom you can share your decision and change process. Someone who is willing to progress through the workbook with you. Choose someone you can trust; someone who will be willing to give you honest feedback. It is helpful if the person has also made a decision to change.

Selecting someone to share the process with can sometimes be stressful in itself. If you do not feel ready to find or choose a partner, begin the process by yourself. You are worth it.

Step 5: If you are not working with a group, set aside time to work through the workbook. Select a day of the week. Choose 30 to 60 minutes on this day. Having a regularly scheduled time is important. Knowing that a special time is available will help to motivate you. Be possessive of this time and do *not* let anything intrude on it. Finally, make sure the setting is quiet and comfortable, and that you will not be disturbed.

If you have a partner, you can use him or her for sharing, support, and encouragement as you work through this workbook. Agree *not* to assume responsibility for each other's issues. Simply be an active listener who provides a "mirror" for the other person as he or she confronts his or her own fears and possibilities. Structured time set aside each week is especially useful for this. If issues or problems arise that you cannot handle or that cause excessive anxiety, seek assistance from another consumer/survivor, a friend, minister, priest, physician, counselor, or therapist. Feedback can be extremely useful in helping you to move ahead and avoid getting stuck. Also, it is OK to seek out assistance at even low levels of distress.

Step 6: As you work through the workbook, you will increase your understanding of your recovery process, of your symptoms and sources of stress, as well as your options for dealing with them. When you feel ready, choose a specific problem or issue you want to work on. For some people the best place to start is with something that is fun or safe.

Others may decide to start with an issue that is causing them some pain. Whatever your choice, be specific. Give yourself permission to deal with one issue at a time.

Step 7: Choose a specific strategy for achieving your goal. Be clear about the steps you must take to deal with the issue you have chosen. If the strategy requires new knowledge or skills, identify where they can be acquired, from whom, and how. Think about the kind of support you will need from people around you and how you can build extra support into your life.

Step 8: Visualize your goal and the steps you plan to take to reach it. Be as detailed as possible. Visualize your plan from beginning to end. Imagine what it will be like for you when you have achieved your goal. Visualization is a very affirming and empowering process.

Step 9: Take action on the steps to reach your goal. Practice. See how it works. Keep at it. Persevere. Remember that it takes a while to change. Find a way to reward yourself for your successes. Remember, success builds on success.

Best wishes on your journey.

Practice Exercise 1.1

𝒴ou will begin exploring and understanding your recovery process with a relaxation exercise. Focusing on your body can be very relaxing. It may even have important physical effects for you such as lowering your heart rate. Stress can cause shallow breathing. Taking a few deep breaths can prepare you for the stresses you may experience while completing this workbook. Relaxation also helps you to let go of what you have been doing during the day and to focus you on the current task.

Find a comfortable position and close your eyes. Begin breathing slowly and deeply—slowly and deeply—all the way into your abdomen—and with each exhalation of your breath let all tension flow out of your body. Continue breathing slowly and deeply—relaxing more and more with each breath.. ❧ Repeat the following phrases to yourself: I am relaxed, I am calm, I am at peace. I am whole—I am whole.. ❧ Now focus your attention on your left foot—tense the muscles in your left foot—then relax your left foot. ❧ Now focus your awareness on your right foot—tense the muscles in your right foot—then relax your right foot. ❧ Now focus on your left calf—tense the muscles in your left calf—then relax your left calf. ❧ Now focus on your right calf—tense the muscles in your right calf—then relax the muscles in your right calf. ❧ Now focus on your left thigh—tense the muscles in your left thigh—then relax your left thigh. ❧ Now focus on your right thigh—tense the muscles in your right thigh—then relax the muscles in your right thigh. ❧ Now focus your attention on your pelvis—tense all the muscles in your pelvis—now relax all the muscles in your pelvis. ❧ Now focus your awareness on your abdomen—tense the muscles in your abdomen—then relax your abdomen. ❧ Now focus on your chest—tense the muscles in your chest—now relax the muscles in your chest. ❧ Now focus on your back—tense the muscles in your back—then relax the muscles in your back. ❧ Now switch to your left upper arm—tense the muscles in your left upper arm—then relax your left upper arm. ❧ Now focus on your right upper arm—tense the muscles in your right upper arm—then relax your right upper arm. ❧ Now focus on your left hand—make a fist and tense the muscles in your left hand—then relax the muscles in your left hand. ❧ Now focus on your right hand—make a fist and tense the muscles in your right hand—then relax your right hand. ❧ Now focus on your neck and shoulders—tense the muscles in your neck and shoulder—then relax your neck and shoulders. ❧ Now focus on your scalp—tense the muscles in your scalp—then relax the muscles in your scalp. ❧ Now focus on your forehead and eyes—tense the muscles in your forehead and eyes—then relax your forehead and eyes. ❧ Now focus on your jaw and mouth—tense the muscles in your jaw and mouth—then relax your jaw and mouth so that all your body is in a state of deep relaxation.

Enjoy the warmth and comfort of deep relaxation. Know that this is an exercise you can come back to at any time by yourself.

[handwritten annotations:]
repeat this throughout exercise
cut?
↑helps to give actual movements to do rather than just tense/relax
Shake out arms or reach up with arms
make a fist with one, stretch out fingers w/ other
roll neck & shrug shoulders

Practice Exercise 1.2

Take a few minutes and complete the following exercise. Think about your responses first, then write them down. When you are finished, go to the next page, and respond to the questions about the exercise.

1. What are three things you did for *yourself* during the previous week?

a.

b.

c.

2. What are three things you can do for *yourself* during the coming week?

a.

b.

c.

Responding to Practice Exercises 1.1 and 1.2

1. What are your own feelings and reactions to *Practice Exercise 1.1 and 1.2?*

2. Authors' comments on *Practice Exercise 1.1 and 1.2*:

When we are feeling overly stressed we tend to forget doing the things that ordinarily take care of us; things that we enjoy and find relaxing. Self-care is often the first thing to go.

Doing things for ourself breaks the cycle of our stress. Interrupting the cycle of our stress is an important stress management strategy.

Doing something different than we are currently doing that is stressful, breaks the cycle of our stress. Even a small interruption, such as going to the bathroom, taking a brief walk, or sitting back and doing a breathing exercise, can break our stress cycle.

Simply eliminating stress can create a vacuum. Fill the vacuum with something enriching. Something you enjoy doing.

Doing things for ourself on a daily basis is a way of gradually building up our stress hardiness. If we feel taken care of, we are in a better position to manage the normal stresses of our life, to take care of other people, or to respond to the demands of our work.

One common result of stress is to feel disconnected from ourself, i.e., from our own needs, wants, feelings, ambitions, and desires. Doing things for ourself helps us to reconnect with ourself; to pay attention to ourself; to listen to what is happening.

Discussion of the importance of "me time" → what are your instructions on an airplane: get your mask on 1st before helping anyone else

Acknowledge that this may not feel right at first
Egosyntonic / Egodystonic

Practice Exercise 1.3

What do you want to get out of th(is workbook)? What would you like to be able to do or to feel after you have completed the workbook? Think about your responses first, then write them down.

Class

Goals worksheet and discussion

a.

b.

Personal Journal/Notes

Personal Journal/Notes

CHAPTER 2 *Recovery*

The Process of Recovery

Recovery is a process of readjusting our attitudes, feelings, perceptions, and beliefs about ourself, others, and life in general. It is a process of self-discovery, self-renewal, and transformation. Recovery is deeply emotional. It transcends the particular trauma itself.

Recovery is a process all people experience at some level, at various times in their life. The more threatening the precipitating event, the more it shakes the roots of who we are and how we experience our life, the more it breaks the connections we took for granted, the more it shatters the dreams and fantasies we hoped for; the deeper and more profound the required recovery process.

Recovery is painful and difficult. It is not something that is usually invited, or even welcomed. It often appears when we are least prepared to deal with it. Yet its outcome can be the emergence of a new sense of self—more real, more vital, more connected to who we really are, more connected to others—and to a greater sense of meaning and purpose in life.

The process of recovery is not linear. It is complex. We move forward and we move backward. We think we have made some gains and then we find we are repeating the same old behaviors. There is a natural resistance to any change process, including the recovery process. The way we are is very persistent. There are few great leaps. People change incrementally. This can be very frustrating. Knowing what the recovery process entails can bring some relief as we experience it.

The process of recovery takes time. Initially, we may feel that time is not on our side, that we will always be where we are now, in a distressing and painful place (Deegan, 1988). Knowing that a major recovery process can take years, while shocking at first, can be a relief. Maybe time is really on our side. There is an end in sight, even if the illness continues. There is a personal outcome that transcends the illness.

We do not know completely how people with psychiatric disability experience the recovery process. We are beginning to understand the course of mental illness over time and some of the factors involved in a person's remaining in one phase or moving on to another (Strauss, Hafez, Lieberman & Harding, 1985), and we are beginning to understand the development of the sense of self in recovery from mental illness (Davidson & Strauss, 1992). While this new awareness has given more hope to people with psychiatric disability, we do not yet know the relationship of the course of the illness to the personal recovery process. However, there are some suggestions of phases of the recovery process (not necessarily linear) that people report experiencing. In addition, there are a number of aspects of the personal recovery process that are emerging from the self-help literature that describe how a person's awareness of him/herself changes over time. Because we are still learning about this process of recovery, both "phases" and "aspects" will be discussed.

Phases of the Recovery Process

Break the class into groups and assign 2 (or 3) phases of recovery to each group. They should read and discuss their phases with each other. Then they should prepare something to present to the class

After each phase is presented, open up for questions & comments.

Shock

The onset of mental illness can be gradual or quite sudden. We may not know what is happening to us. The experience is often confusing and disorganizing. The implications of the illness are devastating to our life, hopes, and dreams. They are too much to grasp.

Denial

It is natural to be unable to accept what is happening. We have lived through crises before. We believe we will weather this one also. It will go away and our life will be normal again. Denial is often the first response to the onset of mental illness. It is a necessary and important, though time-limited, response. Denial serves to cushion the shock of the illness. The illness may be too overwhelming to deal with. Denial gradually gives way to the unrelenting experience of the reality and the persistence of the illness.

There is another type of denial that is often more deliberate. This is the denial that comes from fear of stigma. Fear of the responses of friends, the helping system, or society. We know that stigma is real, and we may not be ready or willing to confront it directly. So we keep our experience to ourself. This is a way of coping.

Depression/Despair/Grieving

Depression is a common reaction to the experience of mental illness. Whether the depression is a direct symptom of the illness or a reactive symptom, it can be dangerous. People who experience serious depression should have an expert health care professional as part of their support system. Depression often leads to despair, i.e., a feeling of hopelessness. If we are supported in our despair by other consumers, friends, and professionals; we can open the door to the grieving process, to the healing of our loss, and to the development of hope.

Depression can continue for a long time. We can get stuck in depression, as in any phase of the recovery process, and feel unable to go on. Getting unstuck is a process of acquiring the support, the information, and the skills we need to deal with what is keeping us stuck. When we are stuck, the tendency of others is to try to move us ahead (Strauss et al., 1985). Like pulling a car out of the mud. Professionals and people close to us are especially threatened by our being stuck because it can make them feel inadequate. What we really need is help in knowing what is currently happening to us and what is getting in our way of moving on. For example, we may simply need time to rest, or to integrate what we have been learning and experiencing. Or we may lack the knowledge, skills, or supports we need to take the next step. When we address these needs, we will naturally move ahead again.

As we move away from depression, we may move into despair and grieving. Since this mourning process is very deeply felt and frightening, depression may feel like a better solution. It is hard to tolerate such strong emotions. This is when the relationship with a helpful person can be especially important: to help us move through the despair and grieving; to fully experience our emotions in a safe way; and to experience the transformation this experience brings about. Despair and grieving will run their course—particularly if we get the personal support we need to sustain ourself during the process.

It's hard for others to hear our despair and grieving. It's often too painful. It's hard to tolerate our pain. Just to be with it and to witness it. To know how awful it is for us. And not to try to take it away. Also, people are so conditioned to act, to do things, that it's hard to just listen and respond and simply be with us. Yet, this is often what we need. To paraphrase the old saying, we may find ourself saying, "Don't just do something, stand there."

Anger

Anger follows on the footsteps of despair and grieving. Anger at the illness which has so devastated us. Anger at the helping system which may have failed and even bruised us at times. Anger at society and its attitudes. Anger at God for not taking better care of us. Anger at parents and friends for not being more helpful. Anger at ourself for not being able to manage our illness.

Our anger is a necessary and important part of the process. Anger is a stimulus to recovery. It is normal and natural. We slowly begin to realize that our anger comes from our strength, our sense of what is right and wrong, our sense of what we need to change, and not from our illness. Our anger is not a "problem" we have, rather it is an asset. It can be frightening, both to ourself and to others. It can be as hard for others to deal with our anger as it is for them to deal with our pain. It can be hard to just hear it, to accept it, to acknowledge its validity, to take it seriously, and not to retaliate. What we need is the support, knowledge, and skills necessary to cope with our anger and to confront whatever sources of our anger we wish to deal with.

In new groups make a poster/collage for each phase.

Acceptance/Hope/Helpfulness

Acceptance, which is an outcome of our despair and grieving, is helped along by the presence of at least one supportive person. Acceptance by others helps us to accept ourself. It is a process that builds gradually, and that is often fragile. Behind our hopelessness is often helplessness. Doing things that are helpful to ourself creates hopefulness, often in small ways that are nevertheless very important, e.g., exercising, reading something we like, spending time with a friend, completing a task we value. These small steps build our confidence and establish a new sense of who we are and what our world is all about. They gradually build a new identity and new meanings. These steps also build an important relationship with another person—someone who believes we count. This gives us the mirroring, feedback, and validation we need.

Coping

Coping is needed when the demands and constraints of our life exceed our resources. So we cope. Coping is learning to live with who we are and what we have to offer the world. Coping is built on acceptance. On seeing ourself directly, without illusions. Coping implies that we know our foundation. What we are building on. Our strengths, our limitations. Our successes, our bruises. Our values and our failures to live up to them. Acceptance relieves some of the pressure of coping. It is OK not to have all the resources. This is normal suffering. It replaces the terror, anguish, and pain we experience when there is no hope and no acceptance—when it is not OK not to have all the resources (Deegan, 1988). Acceptance means that there is nothing that we *need* to do or *should* do. Only what we want to do and are able to do—in the best way that we can.

Advocacy/Empowerment

As our new identity and meanings emerge we support them with increased effort and energy. We become an advocate for ourself. This process is exciting and energizing. We experience ourself differently. We are no longer the same person. The illness may continue, but we have changed. While we may experience our familiar distress with the same old intensity, it does not last as long or happen as frequently. We begin to think, feel, and act in our own interest. We feel more confident and competent.

Our personal advocacy naturally extends to other people who have had experiences similar to ourself. In fact, this is a natural extension of our own healing, i.e., the awareness of our connectedness to others (Bellingham, Cohen, Jones & Spaniol, 1989). Our mutual connectedness. We are not alone in experiencing the effects of our life—nor are others. We experience them in common. We need others and they need us.

Davidson and Strauss (1992) suggest several key aspects of the recovery process based on their longitudinal research with people with psychiatric disability. Their contribution to our understanding of the recovery process has to do with the importance of the sense of self in the recovery process. A sense of self is important to coping and mastery in the living, learning, and working areas of our life. Because one's sense of self is so devastated by mental illness and by stigma, developing a sense of self becomes an important task in the recovery process.

The aspects of a sense of self that Davidson and Strauss (1992) discuss include self-efficacy, self-esteem, and internal locus of control. Key aspects of the recovery of a sense of self are described in the following ways.

Discovering a More Active Self

This is a process of gradually realizing that we can act in our own interest. That we can do things that work, that make our life work, that influence our life. This is a critical awareness in the recovery process. *How* we do this can seem quite minimal to others (e.g., get up on time, keep an appointment, cook a meal), but the discovery that we can influence our life through our own actions can have profound impact on our sense of self. This initial awareness will recur at different times and build up momentum. It is a fragile awareness and may be easily bruised by negative experiences. It is clear that others can be helpful by acknowledging and supporting this process.

Taking Stock of Self

Through additional positive experiences of acting in our own interest we begin to feel more grounded in our new sense of self. While it may continue to feel fragile, we deliberately test out our new found strengths. Confidence builds that our new sense of self exists and is available when we need it. Feedback from others is important during this testing period.

Putting the Self into Action

As our level of confidence in our new sense of self grows, we continue to build our sense of self through personal action and feedback. This is a process of gradually enhancing and further grounding our new sense of self. It is felt as real and available. We can "put our self into action" and further build our sense of self by gradually reclaiming our living, learning, and working life; and confronting negative personal, professional, and societal values, attitudes, and practices.

Appealing to the Self

As our level of confidence grows, we begin to acknowledge more deeply the presence of this stronger sense of self that we can call upon as needed. It becomes a readily available resource for us. While vulnerabilities may continue to exist, we are not so easily bruised by negative life experiences. We feel empowered.

The following exercises will help us to better understand our recovery process, the obstacles to our recovery, and what would be helpful in further promoting our recovery process.

Practice Exercise 2.1   **1.** What does recovery mean to you?

2. What has your recovery process been like for you?

3. What has made the difference for you at various points in your recovery process? What has given you hope?

Practice Exercise 2.2

What are some of the obstacles you are dealing with in your recovery process?

a.

Reason:

b.

Reason:

c.

Reason:

d.

Reason:

_____
Practice Exercise 2.3

What would be helpful to you in improving your recovery process? When you are finished, turn the page and respond to the questions about the exercises.

a.

How?

b.

How?

c.

How?

d.

How?

Responding to Practice Exercises 2.1, 2.2, and 2.3

1. What are your own feelings and reactions to *Practice Exercises 2.1, 2.2, and 2.3?*

2. Authors' comments on *Practice Exercises 2.1, 2.2, and 2.3*:

   It may be hard to experience ourself as being in a process when we seem to be moving so slowly.

   Understanding recovery as a process helps us to cope more effectively with specific stressful events in our life. We know that they will not last forever.

   As we grow in our personal recovery, we identify less with the mental illness and more with other aspects of ourself.

   Our typical reactions to stress are reinforced over time and become very persistent— even if they are no longer wanted.

   Because recovery is not necessarily a linear process, we may be in different phases of our recovery at the same time.

Personal Journal/Notes

Personal Journal/Notes

3 *Increasing Knowledge and Control*

The Impact of Serious Mental Illness

Serious mental illness has a devastating impact on the people who experience it. The language used to describe this impact is important because it has implications for how we view the sources of serious mental illness as well as its impact. Anthony (1993) discusses four major areas of impact on the person (impairment, dysfunction, disability, disadvantage). All four are important in understanding serious mental illness. *Serious mental illness is the result of the unique interaction of combinations of all of these areas, none of which alone provides the complete answer* (Strauss, 1992). These four areas of impact are discussed below, not necessarily in order of occurrence, and presented in Table 3.1 *(page 25)*.

Impairment

The first area of impact is on the physical and psychological level. While we do not know a great deal about the physical aspects of the illness, there is mounting evidence that there is a neurobiological aspect to severe mental illness. The word "impairment" is used to refer to this neurobiological aspect. We know very little about the source of this impairment, whether it is genetic, viral, or some combination of multiple causes. However, the impairment results in the physical and psychological symptoms of the illness, such as hallucinations, delusions, depression, or paranoia. It is important to remember that the occurrence of these symptoms is also influenced by the areas of impact of serious mental illness discussed below. The unique expression of these symptoms is influenced by the psychological structure of the person. As the impairment and its symptoms improve, there is a positive impact on the areas of dysfunction, disability, and disadvantage. The impairment and its symptoms are typically managed by medications and therapy.

The personal experience of the impairment and its symptoms is often referred to by people who are experiencing it as a "loss of self" or a "disruption in the self" (Davidson & Strauss, 1992). We lose our sense of who we are. We feel disconnected from ourself. We do not feel grounded.

Writing exercise:

In what ways has mental illness impacted and changed your life?

Then put up a list for the whole class on the board

While there has been limited success in managing the impairment and its symptoms, we know less about how to help rebuild a disrupted sense of self. Because the assault on the self is the most fundamental impact of mental illness; recovery requires building a functional sense of self that supports our needs, wants, and aspirations and confronts the assaults of stigma (Blanch et al., 1993, in press). Other interventions that have been successful in improving the impairment, as well as our functional sense of self, include coping strategies (Cohen & Berk, 1985; Wiedl & Schottner, 1991), satisfying social relationships (Breier & Strauss, 1984), and self-control of symptoms (Breier & Strauss, 1983).

Dysfunction

The second area of impact is on our ability to carry out the normal activities or tasks of life. The word "dysfunction" is used to describe our inability to perform an activity or task considered normal for a human being. A task might be walking, thinking, talking, making a meal, or going to the beach. The cause of the dysfunction may be the impairment and its symptoms, the side effects of medication, a lack of confidence resulting from a disrupted sense of self, or the effects of stigma. It is important to note that the impairment and its symptoms are not the only potential sources of a dysfunction, and may not be the primary sources. As the dysfunction improves, there is a positive impact on the impairment, the disability, and the disadvantage. As one domain of impact changes, the others appear to change in the same direction. The primary interventions for a dysfunction are assessment, skill training, support, and rehabilitation.

Disability

The third area of impact is on our ability to perform the roles people ordinarily have in life. The word "disability" is used to describe our inability to perform these roles in a manner considered normal for a human being. A disability might be the inability to work, to have a family, to maintain a house or apartment. A disability is a broader concept than a dysfunction because a disability limits our ability to perform larger roles in life. The causes of the disability may be the impairment and its symptoms, a dysfunction, the side effects of medication, a lack of confidence resulting from a disrupted sense of self, or the effects of stigma. As with a dysfunction, it is important to note that the impairment and its symptoms are not the only potential sources of a disability, and may not be the primary sources. The disability impacts negatively on the impairment, the dysfunction, and the disadvantage. It also follows that successful rehabilitation can positively impact on the impairment, the dysfunction, and the disadvantage (Strauss, 1986). The primary intervention for a disability is rehabilitation.

Table 3.1—The Impact of Serious Mental Illness

Stages	Definitions	Examples
1. Impairment	Any loss or abnormality of psychological, physiological, or anatomical structure or function.	Hallucinations, delusions, depression
2. Dysfunction	Any restriction or lack of ability to perform an activity or task in the manner, or within the range considered normal, for a human being.	Lack of: work adjustment skills, social skills, ADL skills
3. Disability	Any restriction or lack of ability to perform a role in the manner, or within the range considered normal, for a human being.	Unemployment, homelessness
4. Disadvantage	A lack of opportunity for an individual that limits or prevents the performance of an activity or the fulfillment of a role that is normal (depending on age, sex, social, cultural factors) for that individual.	Discrimination and poverty

From: Anthony, 1993.

Disadvantage

The fourth area of impact is the lack of opportunity to make a life for ourself. The word disadvantage is used to describe our lack of opportunity which limits or prevents our performing an activity or task, or carrying out our role. The cause of the disadvantage is stigma, discrimination, and poverty. The primary means for confronting disadvantage is personal and group advocacy that influence feelings, beliefs, policy, and legislation. It is important to note that the disadvantage does not simply result from the impairment and its symptoms, from a dysfunction or disability, from the side effects of medication, or from a disrupted sense of self. The disadvantage comes primarily from outside the person, from a society that is unwelcoming because of its biases and prejudices.

[handwritten margin note: unlike the others]

Disadvantage can impact negatively on the impairment, the dysfunction, and the disability. As opportunities become available for the person, there is a positive impact on the impairment, the dysfunction, and the disability. Because all of these areas of impact affect our sense of self, as the areas of impact change for the better or for the worse, our sense of self is influenced for the better or for the worse. As our sense of self becomes stronger, it is less influenced negatively by the impairment, the dysfunction, the disability, and the disadvantage. The primary means for confronting disadvantage is personal and group advocacy that influence feelings, beliefs, policy, and legislation.

The Services of a Recovery-Oriented Mental Health System

A recovery-oriented mental health system has a wide range of services that help people to deal effectively with the impact (impairment, dysfunction, disability, and disadvantage) of a serious mental illness and to build a fulfilling and contributing life for themselves (Table 3.2, *page 27*). While the various services tend to focus on a particular area of impact, there is an interaction effect on other areas. As we change one area of impact, the others are affected in a similar direction.

Treatment

The focus of treatment is on the impairment. The purpose of treatment is to reduce symptoms and to explore and understand feelings, thoughts, values, goals, and roles that enhance recovery. It is important to note that treatment can assist with the direct symptoms of a serious mental illness (hallucinations, delusions, depression, paranoia) as well as with disruption in the sense of self. However, the focus historically has been on reducing symptoms. Hospitalization, medication, and therapy have been the primary treatments.

Rehabilitation

Rehabilitation focuses on the dysfunction and the disability experienced by the people with mental illness. The purpose of rehabilitation is to help people with serious mental illness function in the living, learning, working, and social roles of their lives with the least amount of ongoing professional assistance. Rehabilitation helps with roles such as getting a job, or developing a career direction. Rehabilitation also assists people to reduce dysfunctions by becoming more skillful at activities and tasks that are important in their roles.

As we have stated in the section on areas of impact, there is evidence that rehabilitation also impacts on the impairment, both physically and psychologically (Strauss, 1986). The mind and the body are one. If our life improves we will begin to feel better. This state of well-being has deep implications for our improved physical and psychological functioning. As we become more effective in our roles, our identity is further shaped and our personal meanings become developed and expanded. Our sense of self becomes more integrated and complete. Because serious mental illness impacts so fundamentally on the self, recovery from mental illness requires a rebuilding of the self. Rehabilitation has broad implications for the recovery of the person with serious mental illness.

Crises Intervention

The focus of crises intervention is on problems or barriers to recovery that threaten the person's life or functioning in a dangerous way. The purpose of crises intervention is to help people with serious mental illness survive and get through a dangerous experience in their life. It is important to note that people with serious mental illness prefer

	Goals	Services
Table 3.2—The Goals of a Recovery-Oriented Mental Health System and the Services Required to Meet Them	To reduce symptoms and to explore and understand feelings, thoughts, values, goals, and roles that enhance recovery.	Treatment
	To assist people to be successful and satisfied in chosen roles and settings with the least amount of ongoing intervention by providers.	Rehabilitation
	To deal with dangerous situations that interfere with recovery.	Crises Intervention
	To access services that facilitate recovery.	Case Management
	To advocate for improved services and to eliminate barriers that inhibit recovery.	Rights Protection/ Advocacy
	To promote and support one's own recovery and that of peers with mental illness.	Self-help
	To meet survival needs basic to recovery.	Basic Support
	To enhance quality of life.	Enrichment

Adapted from: Cohen et al., 1988; Anthony, 1993.

to have control over how their crises are handled. This can be done by having the person with a serious mental illness identify in advance and in writing how they want a crises to be handled; for example, who they want notified, how they want to be treated or medicated, where they want the crises treatment to occur, and who they want to treat them. People with serious mental illness want to be dealt with sensitively and consistent with their wishes, even when they are in crises.

Case Management
The focus of case management is on helping people with serious mental illness identify, access, and use the resources they need for their recovery process. Case management should be a collaborative process between the case manager and the person with the mental illness. Client involvement is empowering and furthers the recovery process.

Rights Protection/Advocacy
Rights protection/advocacy focuses on the disadvantages people with serious mental illness experience because of stigma, discrimination, and prejudice. The purpose of rights protection/advocacy is to eliminate barriers and to provide equal opportunities to perform the activities and roles that are normal to human beings.

Self-Help

The focus of self-help is on voluntary mutual aid by peers. The purpose of the self-help might be personal support or it might be focused on social change. Self-help is a growing resource for people with mental illness. Self-help enables people to use their own resources to gain control over their lives. Self-help supports recovery and leads to empowerment.

Basic Support

The focus of basic support is providing the food, clothing, housing, and personal relationships necessary for recovery. Basic support is necessary before people with mental illness can effectively deal with their impairment, dysfunction, disability, and disadvantage. This is most clearly seen when recovery is attempted by someone who is homeless. For example, without basic supports it is hard to deal with our symptoms or getting a job.

Enrichment

The focus of enrichment is on enhancing the quality of life. Enrichment goes beyond meeting basic needs. The purpose of enrichment is to promote creative and enjoyable opportunities for people with mental illness. Enrichment promotes the interests, abilities, and capacities of people with mental illness.

The Values of a Recovery-Oriented Mental Health System

*V*alues are the motivating force of a recovery-oriented mental health system. They are its foundation and its purpose for existing as a system. The values drive the system and all its components (Table 3.3).

Empowerment

Coping refers to a person's efforts to manage internal and external demands and constraints that exceed his/her resources. Empowerment is an important outcome of a successful coping process. Even small successes at coping can lead to this feeling of empowerment. Empowerment is the realization that we have the right, the ability, and the resources to determine what our needs and wants are and to pursue them. Feeling empowered means feeling that we are worthwhile and that we count; that we are real, have choices, can make decisions, can trust our feelings, respect our strengths and limitations, can call on others for assistance; that there is more to us than our illness.

Empowerment is an attitude and a feeling that is often difficult to maintain. It is vulnerable to disappointments and to setbacks. Yet, it grows with our successes and with the support of others.

	Value	Description
Table 3.3—The Values of a Recovery-Oriented Mental Health System	Empowerment	Creating a personal vision and having the confidence to move toward it.
	Client choice	People can make their own decisions about how to lead their life.
	Client involvement	Participating in the processes by which decisions are made that affect one's life.
	Community-focus	Building on existing connections.
	Client strengths	Watering the flowers and not the weeds.

Adapted from: Anthony, 1993.

Awareness of our own worth and value.

Individuals are important. We count. We can have an impact on our own life and the lives of others. Our potential for impact in our work and personal life increases as our acknowledgment of our own worth and value increases. Personal crises often confront long-held beliefs and values. The resulting crises in meaning, when worked through, can lead to a deepening of our values and beliefs.

Examples from the self-help literature:

Acknowledging how far I have come.

Don't compare myself with others.

Life always offers me another chance.

Speaking about my illness only when I am asked. Not volunteering information.

Attending classes, while difficult at times, forced me to think about something other than myself.

Learned about "boundaries" and their importance in all relationships, and how to set them and change them when needed.

Gave up the grandiose ideas that I could "save society," and concentrated on seeking inner peace and harmony by being a constructive influence with my significant others, peers, and professional colleagues.

Chose to consciously replace fears with "faith," knowing that the mind cannot hold two simultaneous thoughts. Whenever fears come up I now acknowledge them, experience them, talk about them, take action, if necessary, and create an affirmation of faith.

I have learned not to talk to myself or to my voices when others are near by.

Client Choice

Client choice means that people with mental illness have the right to choose the direction and the means of their own recovery. It means that at every point in the process the person with the mental illness has the right to make the decision. Because people may at times be unable to make the decision needed, it is helpful to have a mutually negotiated agreement in advance that points out how they want to be helped when they are unable to decide for themselves. Rushing people to a decision or taking over their lives without their approval damages the recovery process.

Client choice supports client responsibility. Asking people to be responsible without giving them the choice to be responsible, may promote surface agreement and hidden rebellion.

Client Involvement

Client involvement means that people have the right to be involved in decisions that affect their lives. People with mental illness should be involved in the planning, implementation and evaluation of their own recovery process. Involvement is empowering. It puts the person with the mental illness in charge of his or her own recovery.

Community-Focus

Community-focus means that there is an emphasis on building and using existing connections. The purpose of this focus is to have the person with the mental illness connect with resources and supports that are familiar and available. Uprooting people from their natural resources and supports adds another layer of adjustment to what is already a very distressing experience.

Client Strengths

While the experience of serious mental illness can be debilitating, a person frequently retains many active strengths, as well as hidden strengths, that can be called upon with adequate knowledge, skill training and support. Mental health treatment has traditionally focused on the illness and reducing symptoms of the illness. The many strengths of people have been frequently ignored. Recovery is supported by acknowledging and building on strengths.

Personal Journal/Notes

Personal Journal/Notes

Hmwk # 4

Continue journaling
Read at least 2 of Moe Armstrong's poems in
   Preparation for meeting him next week.

Hmwk # 5

Continue Journaling
Write your own definition of stress

CHAPTER 4 *Managing Life's Stresses*

Symptoms of Stress

Stress is a common human experience. We all experience stress every day in our lives. At times, stress may be helpful because it motivates us in some important ways. It may help us to complete a task or to rise above and beyond our usual capacities. However, when our stress becomes distressful, it interferes with our ability to manage our life and to promote our recovery process. Then, we begin to experience our stress as a burden.

People with psychiatric disability experience stress in the living, learning, and working areas of their lives. While these sources of stress are common to all people, the presence of direct and reactive symptoms of mental illness (often referred to as positive and negative symptoms in the mental health literature) can make stress more difficult to cope with. Direct symptoms come from the illness itself and may include anxiety, hallucinations, delusions, and depression. Reactive symptoms are side-effects of the illness, its treatment, or the environment; and may include apathy, alienation, demoralization, low energy, and low self-esteem. For example, reactive symptoms may result from experiences of discrimination and stigma. Coping with these direct and reactive symptoms, and with the normal stresses of life, is a task that confronts people with psychiatric disability in their recovery process.

Lazarus and Folkman (1984) have stated that people's reactions to potential stressors are a function of their conscious and unconscious appraisal of how threatening a particular internal or external stressor is to them. This appraisal is affected by the information, skills, and supports we possess to deal with stressful situations. If we perceive that a stressor will exceed our resources, we will begin to experience physical and emotional stress reactions. The length and intensity of these reactions will depend on how serious we perceive the threat to be. Increasing the range of options for dealing with potentially stressful situations can increase the ability of people with psychiatric disability to cope with internal and external stressors.

We have written this section of the workbook as a resource for people with psychiatric disability to help them prevent, eliminate, or cope with the stressors in their lives that interfere with their recovery process. We believe that it is never too late to turn our life around. Looking at how we currently experience and cope with stressful situations can be an important first step. For example, we can begin to understand some of the connections between our distress and its causes. Distress does not just appear from nowhere. It has identifiable internal and external causes. We may find it difficult and painful to explore the connection between how we are feeling and functioning now, and what has led up to it. Yet there are connections; whether recent or remote, simple or complex. Once we become aware of these connections, we can begin the process of exploring, understanding, and acting in order to prevent, interrupt, or manage stressful situations. This is what coping is all about: acknowledging symptoms of stress, exploring their causes and meanings, and intervening to relieve them.

States of well being also have causes. This knowledge can open up the exciting possibility of promoting and increasing our own well-being. The process of identifying and building on positive internal and external resources can help us to build a fulfilling, meaningful, and contributing life that goes beyond merely managing stressful situations. The field of psychology is beginning to explore what leads to personal empowerment, higher levels of functioning, peak performance, and well being, and what we can do to begin promoting that shift in our own life. Although we may never be able to leave the coping process completely, simply coping with our life can become dull and boring. The exercises in this chapter will help us to promote our own well-being and to enhance our recovery process.

Levels of Stress

All people have a typical general physical and emotional response to stress (Table 4.1, *page 37*). However, no one person has all of the symptoms, nor do people experience the same symptom in the same way. Stress can be viewed as having three levels:

First Degree: At this level the symptoms are mild. They may be occasional and short-lived. What we ordinarily do to take care of ourself removes the symptom. We may distract ourself, rest for a while, take a break from our work, or simply relax. Whatever we do is usually successful, and we can return to what we need to do.

Second Degree: When this level occurs our symptoms are more regular, last longer, and are more difficult to eliminate. What we ordinarily do to manage our stress does not work as well. After a night's sleep we may still be tired. Even a weekend may not be enough to eliminate our symptoms. We find that it takes extra effort to take care of ourself.

Third Degree: At this level our symptoms are continuous. We may develop physical or psychological problems such as ulcers or depression. What we ordinarily do to take care of ourself seems useless for dealing with our symptoms. Even medical and/or psychological assistance may not bring quick relief. Existential and philosophical concerns may arise. We may question the value of our work, relationships, or even life itself.

Our symptoms are often our first sign that something is not going well for us. Acknowledging and accepting responsibility for our symptoms is a first step in managing stress in our life. Acknowledgment involves recognition and acceptance of the content, feelings, and meanings of our experiences, as well as our role and that of our environment in producing these experiences. Achieving this awareness may be difficult at times. If we have been denying our symptoms or their impact on our life we may find ourself resisting this new awareness.

The earlier we can acknowledge our symptoms the easier it is to interrupt them and to begin to understand and deal with their causes. Awareness of symptoms provides us with an early warning signal for interrupting the process that leads to excessive stress. The process that leads to stress is often more disruptive than the content of our stress. The content of our stress frequently changes, whereas the process that leads to stress remains the same. Understanding how we become stressed, will prepare us to interrupt or prevent it.

Ignoring our symptoms, "toughing it out," or waiting until the symptoms build up and force us to deal with them, are all ways we keep doing what hasn't worked. Denial can be pervasive. The earlier we can interrupt our stress process, the easier it is to try something else. Identifying and coping with symptoms at earlier and earlier levels of intensity is an important step toward managing stress. As we get good at identifying our symptoms, we can begin to interrupt our cycle of stress. We can even begin to anticipate it and prevent it. We become "wise" about ourself.

Symptoms that are persistent often have an important role to play in our life. We have come to need them, either in our awareness or out of our awareness. Trying to remove a symptom that we are invested in for some reason brings about a great deal of resistance. The harder we work to eliminate them, the stronger they seem to become. Understanding how our symptoms serve our interests may be an important step in managing our stress. This level of self-awareness is often very painful because of the feelings it brings with it. Special support from a friend or therapist is especially helpful in this situation. It isn't necessary to do this all by ourself.

Why Managing Life's Stresses Is Important

1. Stress can be physically and psychologically harmful. Susceptibility to intense negative feelings, illness, and accidents increase when stress increases. We can not maintain ourselves indefinitely under high levels of stress. The accumulation of unresolved stresses tends to wear down our body and our mind. It interferes with our recovery process.

2. Our stress is potentially harmful to others. We may become more critical of them. We may show them less concern. We may even physically or emotionally abuse them because we are so frustrated or angry.

3. Stress reduces the amount of energy available for constructive problem solving, creative and innovative work, sharing and cooperating with others, and enjoying life. We have a fixed amount of energy. If our energy is being used up by excessive stress, we are short-changing ourself and others.

Benefits of Managing Life's Stresses

can do more using coping energy for something else

1. The release of surprising personal capacities to create, produce and recover. The energy we have been putting into coping can be transformed into a creative force.

confidence ? control

2. Increased confidence in changing ourself and our world. Increased ability to manage our life and our environment.

helping others

3. Through personal example we may encourage our friends, families, and others to promote their abilities and utilize their full capacities.

General Stress Response

Stress: Stress is a normal part of a healthy life. It is a non-specific response of the body to a demand or constraint. It does not matter whether the demand or constraint is pleasant or unpleasant. If it is intense or prolonged it may become distressful.

Stimulus: Anything that may result in stress.

- *Internal:* Physical, emotional, intellectual or spiritual aspects of ourself, e.g., illness, disability, conflicts, attitudes, memories, beliefs, expectations, meaning, purpose.

- *External:* Positive or negative events

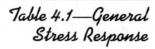

Table 4.1—General Stress Response

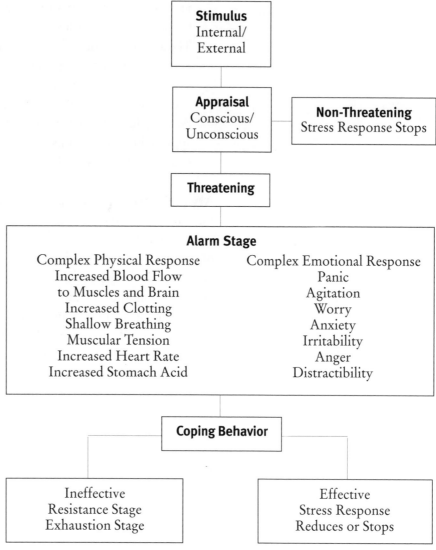

Adapted from: Lazarus, 1976; Selye, 1974; Shaffer, 1982; Spaniol, 1993.

Appraisal:

- Our continuous re-evaluations of the demands and constraints of our internal and external environment and of our options and resources for managing them.

- The degree to which we experience psychological stress is determined by our evaluation of what is at stake and our coping resources and options.

- A stimulus becomes a stressor only when our mind identifies it as such and as long as our mind continues to identify it as such. Thus, our perception of threat can change over time and influence the course of our stress reaction. It is the meanings we place on our internal and external experiences from moment to moment that determine our physical and psychological reactions.

Stimulus

↓

Appraisal

Threatening   Nonthreatening

↓   ↓

Alarm Stage   stress stops

↓

Coping Behavior

Ineffective   Effective

↓   ↓

stress accumulates   stress reduces

wear down/burn out   or stops

crisis may result

- Our mind is the trigger to the stress response. Understanding the relationship between our mind and our stress response is fundamental to managing stress.
- The appraisal process may be conscious or unconscious. If our perception of threat represents an unconscious fear, then the stress reaction of the alarm stage may be especially frightening and out of control. We may be less likely to know why we are reacting and what we are reacting to. However, when the appraisal process is conscious we are better able to identify the source of the stress and to react appropriately.

Alarm Reaction: If our appraisal concludes that the stressor is threatening, a complex series of physical and emotional reactions occur. The intensity and duration of these reactions relate to the level of threat we perceive. As long as we perceive a threat, we will continue to experience increased tension. The alarm reaction may even become a conditioned response to situations we perceive as threatening, either consciously or unconsciously. As we change our appraisal of the stressor, there may be a lag in the change in our reaction. Our tendency to remain the way we are is very strong. This may require living with some distress or discomfort while we are changing. We can reduce the frequency and duration of the alarm reaction but not eliminate it entirely. We maintain a vulnerability to internal and external events we once appraised as threatening.

In addition to the immediate physical and emotional reactions to stress, there are intellectual and spiritual reactions that may occur if the stress continues. The intellectual reactions can include complaining, rationalizing, "awfullizing," and exaggerating the event. The spiritual reactions relate to loss of meaning or purpose, and a sense of disconnectedness and alienation.

Coping: Coping reflects our efforts to manage internal and external demands and constraints that exceed our resources. There are four basic and often overlapping approaches to coping. The extent to which we are skillful in using these approaches determines the extent to which we can mediate both our appraisal of the situation and our coping with it. Our level of coping skills reflects our stress hardiness.

- *Physical:* Fitness, exercise, relaxation techniques, nutrition, diet.

- *Emotional:* Acknowledging feelings and resolving conflicts, feeling good about ourself, making a commitment, feeling challenged, feeling in charge, having a supportive relationship.

- *Intellectual:* Being open to new ideas; problem-solving and decision-making activity; focusing thoughts; redefining problems in more useful terms, e.g., acknowledging that we cannot or need not control all situations; developing resources; planning.

- *Spiritual:* Finding meaning or a larger purpose in ourself, others, or our environment.

Resistance: We mobilize to fight the stressor through coping. If mobilization is inadequate the resistance stage begins. If the resistance stage lasts too long we may begin to feel depleted. Long-term resistance implies that we are not able to solve the problem or to cope effectively. Physical, emotional, intellectual, and spiritual symptoms may increase during this stage. It is the accumulation of stressors rather than a single major stressor that tends to wear us down. With a major stressor, it may be easier to focus our coping responses and to recover.

Exhaustion: When our resources are depleted, we will experience exhaustion. Exhaustion is commonly known as "burn-out." As we reach higher levels of burn-out we become vulnerable to physical, emotional, intellectual, and spiritual breakdown. On the other hand, if the coping response is effective, the alarm reaction will reduce or cease.

Practice Exercise 4.1

What are three of your symptoms of stress. What happens to you when you feel under stress. Include at least one physical symptom.

1.

2.

3.

Practice Exercise 4.2

How do you currently deal with your stress symptoms?

Ineffective strategies

1.

2.

3.

Effective strategies

1.

2.

3.

Responding to Practice Exercises 4.1 and 4.2

1. What are your own feelings and reactions to *Practice Exercises 4.1 and 4.2?*

2. Authors' comments on *Practice Exercises 4.1 and 4.2:*

Symptoms are messengers. They are clues that tell us when we need to stop what we are doing, to interrupt our typical stress-inducing process, and to try something else. If we have been ignoring our symptoms, we may need to practice refocusing our attention on how we feel when we are stressed.

Symptoms are also guides that can lead us to understanding how we become stressed. Identifying how we become stressed is important in managing our stress.

Our symptoms are also our solutions. They develop from our first attempts to mobilize our body and our mind to combat a stressor. They are often not very helpful solutions to what we are facing, but they have been our best way up to now to deal with the sources of our stress.

Acknowledging that symptoms have been solutions also acknowledges that we have tried to deal with our stressors. While it is painfully true that "If something doesn't work, we keep doing it," we can learn to try something else. We don't have to accept the current solution because we can learn to develop more helpful solutions.

The way we are is our best solution to life as we have experienced it up to now.

Sources of Stress

There are many sources of stress for people with a psychiatric disability (Table 4.2). Some of these sources are within individuals and some are within the environment. For example, the illness itself is a major source of stress. Learning to accept and to cope with the illness and its symptoms takes a great deal of energy. Other common sources of stress are the negative attitudes and practices people with psychiatric disability encounter in their living, learning, and working lives (Deegan, 1992). Negative attitudes and practices are intrusive. They provoke many feelings, including shame and anger.

The accumulation of small stressors is often more distressing than a large stressor. This may seem contrary to popular belief, but it is true. Large stressors are difficult to avoid and demand our immediate attention. Small stressors can be easily put off or ignored until they build up and overwhelm us.

Non-judgmental awareness is important in dealing with stressors. Identify how you are. Don't judge or compare yourself to others. Discounting ourself for "not doing it right" is not helpful. It is important not to be hard on ourself. This only adds to our stress. Sometimes finding out what we gain by our stress or what we have to give up to let go of our stress can be helpful. Eliminating stressors may actually increase our stress temporarily because we can no longer ignore what the stressor had allowed us to avoid. It is important to build some supports into our life while we actively eliminate stressors.

The purpose of this section is to look at some of your own personal and environmental sources of stress and how you currently cope with them.

Table 4.2— Internal/External Sources of Stress

1. Changes in our life
2. Losses in our life
3. Stigma (negative attitudes, beliefs, and practices)
4. Personal beliefs
5. Unresolved conflicts
6. Loss of control over our life
7. Personal lifestyle
8. Innate biological vulnerability
9. Lack of fitness
10. Unwillingness to make a commitment
11. Lack of connectedness
12. Lack of meaning or purpose

Practice Exercise—4.3 List three things that are causing you stress.

1.

2.

3.

Practice Exercise—4.4 **H**ow do you currently cope with your sources of stress?

Ineffective strategies

1.

2.

3.

Effective strategies

1.

2.

3.

Practice Exercise—4.5 **W**hat are three key ways that you contribute to your own stress? What do you do (or not do) that leads you to feel stressed?

1.

2.

3.

Practice Exercise—4.6 $\mathcal{H}$ow do you currently cope with how you contribute to your own stress?

Ineffective strategies

1.

2.

3.

Effective strategies

1.

2.

3.

Responding to Practice Exercises 4.3 to 4.6

1. What are your own feelings and reactions to *Practice Exercises 4.3 to 4.6*?

2. Authors' comments on *Practice Exercises 4.3 to 4.6*:

We are not alone in how we experience our life. Others have similar experiences. We can learn from one another.

Having a disability is not a problem. It is a given. Problems arise in how we cope with that disability and how we cope with the many social and interpersonal barriers we have to deal with daily.

If something doesn't work we often keep doing it anyway. Why not try something else instead? The more options we have for managing stress, the more successful we are likely to be.

Coping Strategies

Slowing Down and Relaxing

There are three "slowing down and relaxing" coping strategies that we will present in this section. They are "pacing," "learning to feel and sense rather than think about a problem," and "learning to say no and to set limits on our commitments."

1. **Pacing.** Learn to pace ourself. Become aware of our daily and monthly rhythms. Acknowledge to ourself when our energy is low and when it is high. Structure our activities in ways that acknowledge our energy flow. Brief breaks help to restore our energy. Learn to focus attention on what we are currently doing from moment to moment. Energy focused on a specific task can slow the body and the mind, increase creativity, and save energy. Rushing from task to task or allowing ourself to become "scattered" in our life and work will increase our stress levels and use up our resources. Focused attention is enhanced when we are able to let go of even thinking about past or future activities.

"Pacing our mind" means acknowledging how our mind tends to wander out of the present. We can learn to gently refocus our mind back to our current activity. An unfocused mind or one that is busy with a lot of unwanted or unnecessary thoughts is a major source of energy drain. Daily meditation or other focusing exercises build our capacity to focus our attention on the present. We can train our mind to focus on what we want it to focus on.

We can also train our mind to resist negative or intrusive thoughts. Negative and intrusive thoughts are distortions in thinking. A distortion in thinking is a misperception. We may not see the misperception because we have come to believe it as real. Whatever the source of our distortions, the distortions are often accompanied by distressing feelings and emotions. These distressing feelings and emotions are one way by which we can identify our distortions. We can learn to challenge our distortions in a number of ways. One way is by substituting them with more helpful and hopeful thoughts *(Practice Exercise 4.8)*. Another way is by developing positive affirmations that acknowledge our many strengths *(Practice Exercise 4.9)*.

Further strategies for managing negative and intrusive thoughts:

a. *Quieting the mind.*

- *Medication:* Many people find medication helpful in quieting the mind. In some cases, medication by itself does not fully quiet the mind and additional strategies are needed.

- *Focusing on sensation rather than thinking:* Music, exercise, yoga, and other activities that focus on sensations in the body can quiet the mind. Some people find activity more relaxing than slowing-down exercises such as meditation.

- *Meditation:* Many people find meditation helpful. Meditation quiets the mind by focusing our attention on the sensation of air as it enters and leaves our nostrils or by focusing on a particular object or sound.

b. **Stopping the thoughts before they take over.** We can become skillful at stopping thoughts before they take over our mind. Some people find simply saying "no" to the thoughts and focusing on some other activity helpful in stopping them. Other people find that by pulling on a rubber band on their wrist they can stop the thought. The earlier we say "no," the easier it is to stop the thoughts. Once the thought gathers momentum it is harder to stop.

c. **Interrupting the thoughts before they become overwhelming.** If the thoughts have already begun to take over our mind we can still interrupt them. In order to manage them we must break the cycle of their energy. We can tell ourself that if I am anxious or obsessive, this must be a distortion. We can check out the thoughts with another person. We can distract ourself by focusing on another activity. Do not "kick" yourself for getting caught up in a negative thought again. "Kicking ourself" is another way of building up negative energy. Be gentle on yourself. Simply refocus your energy on something else.

d. **Setting aside time for the thoughts.** Some people find having a special time for their thoughts helpful. Having ten minutes a day to have our thoughts allows us to more easily set them aside outside of that time. We know we have a time for them. This special time should be a time when we have energy. It should not be a time when we tend to be tired because we are more vulnerable at that time. We should not lie down during this time, but sit up erect—with attention. Some people prefer to pace. It should not be before a meal or after a meal. It should not be when we first get up in the morning or before we go to bed. The time should be strictly limited to ten minutes per day. We can move to every other day, every third day, etc., as we get better at this.

e. **Accepting that the thoughts are there and focusing on other activities.** At times we cannot completely get rid of the thoughts. However, we can still distract ourselves even though the thoughts may still remain. They can be very persistent. Just acknowledge their presence and move on to something else.

Examples from the self-help literature:

Not brooding—finding a way to get away from it. Changing my pace or refocusing my energy. By achieving small goals I increase my self-confidence.

Establishing a reasonable routine, a slower pace, and a calm atmosphere. Setting up a schedule for myself provided a structure for everyday living.

Scheduling "down time" at the end of the day—about 30 minutes to an hour of quiet before bedtime to read, write in my diary, lounge in a tub of hot water.

Keeping a notebook with a calendar and addresses and phone numbers, and a running list of tasks to be accomplished—reminded me of what was important.

When I have been tested emotionally or stretched beyond my limits, I write a letter focusing on all that's good in my life. Writing seems to empty my mind of information that interferes with action and helps to organize me.

If I have a great deal to accomplish in a short period of time I write down the tasks that need to be accomplished and list them from most important to least important.

Learned to monitor my energies and not overdo or over tire.

I have had to plan the use of my time. The structure of a predictable daily schedule makes life easier.

Making lists organizes my thoughts.

The following exercises will help us to further understand and to practice "pacing" ourself. *Practice Exercise 4.7* will help us to see how we currently organize our day. We will look at how we might organize our day differently to make better use of our energy. *Practice Exercise 4.8* will help us to identify the negative thoughts that are using up our energy. We will learn how to rephrase these negative thoughts in a positive way. Negative thoughts drain our energy. Positive thoughts give us more energy. *Practice Exercise 4.9* will help us to identify positive aspects of ourself. We can come to believe in these positive aspects of ourself, and remind ourself of them when we are feeling down. Each of these exercises will help us to "pace" our body and our mind more effectively.

Practice Exercise 4.7   **1.** List your activities for an ordinary day.

Morning

Afternoon

Evening

2. How can you organize your day differently to make better use of your energy?

Practice Exercise 4.8   **Identifying Negative Thoughts**   **Rephrasing Thoughts in a Positive Way**

1. Negative thought: Positive thought:

   Feelings associated with   Feelings associated with
   the negative thought: the positive thought:

2. Negative thought: Positive thought:

   Feelings associated with   Feelings associated with
   the negative thought: he positive thought:

3. Negative thought: Positive thought:

   Feelings associated with   Feelings associated with
   the negative thought: the positive thought:

Practice Exercise 4.9 **Affirmations**

1. List positive things about yourself. Both things you believe about
   yourself and positive things others have said about you.

Catherine
Great listener, v. deep thinker
Sweet + sensitive
meek
Always smiley ☺

Amy
so smart (v. caring
great teacher
nice smile
Seem comfortable in
"your own skin"
(confident)

2. Carry this list with you. When you are feeling besieged by
   negative or intrusive thoughts read the list to yourself.

2. Learn to feel and to sense rather than to think about a problem.
Thinking is often the only solution we use to problem-solve. It often
takes the form of worrying—a thinking solution. Thinking triggers thinking. It also tends to ward off feelings and emotions. Experiencing emotions is helpful in resolving problems. The more we can experience the
emotions, the more we can change. The process of emotional experiencing results in feeling resolved about a problem.

Instead of thinking, try feeling and sensing an issue or concern without thinking about it. Feeling means getting in touch with our emotions.
Sensing means getting in touch with the emotional and physical tensions
in our body. Our emotional and physical tensions are important clues to
what is happening within us. Thinking can switch our attention from
these important processes. Take a half hour in a quiet place to experience
feelings and sensations without thinking. See what images emerge that
give clues to current concerns. Imagery is a helpful way to tap the emotions. This "focusing effort" can be a scary and draining process when
first experienced. With time we will become more comfortable with the
process and will trust the wisdom of our emotions and body.

It is important to recognize that we can experience and express our
feelings *without acting on them*. It is often more difficult, and more
courageous, to express our feelings than to act on them. We may be
frightened by our feelings because we believe they will get out of control
if we express them. Yet we can experience and express affection without
acting on it. We can experience and express anger without acting on it.
Practicing experiencing and expressing our emotions in a safe environment can help us to feel more confident in ourself.

Examples from the self-help literature:

*Learning to recognize and express my feelings. Finding useful ways to vent
my feelings. Don't let the feelings build up.*

Learning to cry when I feel sad. To express my emotions naturally.

Learning how to say no, I can't, I don't want to.

*Interviewed and sought out paid professionals who were willing to hear
and process pain, anger, and grief as many times as were necessary in a
shame-free environment.*

Learning to laugh about my experiences.

Refining my ambitions.

*Used creative materials such as clay, colored pens and paper,
art materials, fabrics, etc., to express feelings that I could not
verbalize.*

*Used therapeutic hobbies, such as swimming and gardening, to relieve
tension.*

*Moved out of destructive relationships and avoided non-nurturing places
and events. I can be over stimulated by too much sensory input, so I stay
out of places like shopping malls. I choose to be with nurturing, non-sham-
ing people in healthy environments.*

I have come to accept that taking medication is important to my staying out of the hospital.

Becoming more in touch with feelings of anger and rage, and my aggression in general, and being more in the present, helped me to deal with my sensory overload.

I had the courage to face up to my problems, to come to terms with my thoughts and feelings, to do what I needed to do even when I wasn't feeling well.

Mourning the dreams I had that I wasn't able to realize. I've seen friends pass me by in their careers and in the growth of their families.

I will check my paranoid thoughts out with someone I trust to get feedback and to calm myself down.

My support group has been a very practical resource in accepting and dealing with my mental illness.

I make a list of the names of all the emotions I can think of. This helps me to focus my attention on feelings, and gives me some control over them.

If I am fearful, I sing or chant mantras or songs to myself: a prayer, a song, anything that I am very familiar with, to keep my mind from being distracted by fear.

I empowered myself by registering to vote. This gave me an identity as a citizen, and some measure of control over my own fate. Involvement with the arts, either passive (e.g., reading a poem) or active (e.g., painting a scene) helps to ground my feelings.

I work with anger, not against it. Anger, like any other negative emotion (lust, resentment, envy, covetousness, fear, anxiety, hatred, rage, frustration) cannot "belong" to anyone, any more than the rain belongs to someone. I know that these emotions are simply part of the ambience, and if allowed to run their course will change into something else. So as the voice teacher says, I work on my break.

My apathy comes simply from the refusal to feel my negative feelings. When I block my negative feelings, I block my positive feelings, and stagnation, followed by exhaustion, is the result.

Once my positive and negative emotions start to flow, the manic energy can become so potent that magic is possible. I must decide for myself whether or not to use these magical powers. I remind myself that yogis are enjoined not to exercise the siddhis, as these powers are called, in order to go beyond them to a higher, purer state.

Practice Exercise 4.10

1.   What is something you are glad about?

2.   What is something you are angry about?

3.   What is something you are sad about?

4.   What is something you are scared of?

5.   Who is someone you could express the above feelings to? Name that person or persons.

3. Learn to say "no" and to set limits on our commitments.
Think of our current activities and commitments. Decide which ones are really not necessary and possibly not even consistent with our own values and interests. Begin to eliminate them from our personal and work life. Take some time to acknowledge our own values and interests. Do not accept any new commitments unless they are absolutely necessary. Refocus our energies in directions that take better care of us.

Process for Setting Limits:

1. Finding support for ourself as we set the limits.

2. Being firm about what we do not like.

3. Being clear about what we do like.

4. Helping others to be clear about what they want.

5. Being clear to others concerning what we are able or willing to do.

6. Acknowledging our competencies and not going beyond them.

7. Knowing our limits and not waiting to be pushed over the edge.

8. Knowing that structure can communicate caring.

9. Caring enough not to let another person do something that is harmful to him/herself or to others and encouraging him/her to do things that are in their own best interest.

10. Negotiating what we will and will not do.

11. Living with the upset our limits cause and getting through it.

12. Having another point out when we are going beyond our limits. Someone we trust.

13. You don't have to say yes/no right away, you can take some time.

Practice Exercise 4.11   **1.** Describe a situation in which you want to say "no" or to set some limits.

2. What would you like to do differently? Be clear about what you want and don't want.

3. What is most likely to go wrong? How can you deal with this?

4. What is likely to go right?

Physical Wellness

Definition

Physical wellness involves cardiovascular endurance, flexibility and strength, and physical activity. It also includes good nutrition, medical self-care and disease prevention, and safety behaviors. We are better able to work, play, and enjoy life if we keep active; eat and drink sensibly; and learn to prevent, treat, and recover from illness. We can have a major impact on our health by becoming better informed about health choices and behaviors.

The Relationship of Improved Physical Wellness to Recovery

A person's physical wellness is very important when recovering from mental illness. Increasing fitness, eating well, and sleeping regular hours can increase our tolerance of the daily hassles and stress that are encountered in taking back control of our life. Exercising regularly and eating well can help us feel better about our body which in turn can help us feel better about ourself and our life.

Often people who have experienced a psychiatric illness have been subject to taking medications that may help their symptoms, but have side effects (enormous weight gain, fatigue, food cravings) that deplete personal levels of physical wellness.

Recent research (Skrinar, Hutchinson & Williams, 1992) has studied the impact of increased physical fitness on mental illness. The results have significant implications for the recovery process from mental illness. As people became more fit by exercising regularly, they felt less depressed, their self-esteem rose, their moods improved, their symptoms decreased in intensity, and their level of activity in their lives increased.

Taking control of our physical wellness by increasing our fitness, eating sensibly, and practicing safe social behaviors and medical self-care is very empowering and can be an important support in our recovery from mental illness.

Dimensions of Physical Wellness

- Cardiovascular endurance (a strong, healthy heart)
- Flexibility and strength
- Physical activity
- Sensible nutrition
- Medical self-care and disease prevention
- Safe social behaviors

Cardiovascular endurance: is the ability of the heart, blood vessels, and blood to carry oxygen to the cells. Cardiovascular endurance can be improved through aerobic exercise. Aerobic exercise is any activity that pumps more oxygen to our heart, muscles, and lungs. Examples include: brisk walking, jogging, swimming, cycling, rowing machine, skating, dancing.

Flexibility and strength: refers to our muscles and joints and their movement through their full range of motion and to the force a muscle can produce in one motion. Improving our flexibility and strength can be achieved through gentle stretching, weight lifting, and aerobic exercises (i.e. brisk walking).

Physical activity: is any activity where we use our body in a positive, productive manner that increases our heart rate. Increasing our level of physical activity is important if we choose to improve our health, prevent disease, and live longer and better. It can be as simple as using the stairs instead of the elevators, getting off the subway or bus one stop prior to our own and walking the rest of the way. It is important to remember that anyone can achieve fitness, no matter our age. We do not need to be a professional athlete to be fit.

The American College of Sports Medicine recommends that people exercise a minimum of three times a week for at least thirty minutes at a time. Exercise should be enjoyable as well as good for us. Include variety in our exercise program or exercise with friends. Different activities and companionship can help bolster our perseverance and satisfaction with an exercise routine.

Another way to include more physical activity in our life is to use a community resource. Often Adult Education Centers offer exercise programs that are affordable and accessible. Local YMCA/YWCAs, community colleges, and high schools provide potential opportunities for swimming or group activities such as volleyball, basketball, and softball.

Sensible nutrition: An important part of recovery is acknowledging that we are worth taking good care of ourselves. Eating well and taking responsibility for our bodies is empowering. Recovering from mental illness requires rebounding from the negative side effects of medication, depression, and social isolation; including weight gain, low self-esteem, lethargy, weakness, intestine and bowel problems, and skin problems. Eating sensibly can have a profound impact on our recovery from a psychiatric illness. We can lose weight, feel and look better, and have more energy and strength to participate in our life the way we want to. One barrier to eating a balanced diet are myths about food and eating behaviors that over the years we have learned are just not true.

Common Myths about Food

- Potatoes, rice, pasta are fattening.

- Skipping meals shrinks our stomach so then we have a smaller appetite and will lose weight.

- We need to eat more during the winter to keep warm.

- Dieting is the only way to lose weight.

- Natural sugar is bad for us.

- We need to eat a lot of meat to stay strong.

- Don't exercise for one hour after eating.

Sensible Guidelines about Food

1. *Eat three meals a day.* The secret to permanent weight control is not a diet but an eating and exercise management plan that we have for the rest of our life. Skipping meals actually causes weight gain because our body's metabolism slows down in response to the lack of food.

2. *Eat a variety of foods, in moderation.* Fruits, vegetables, pasta, rice, whole grain breads, low fat/no fat dairy products, and lean meats (poultry and fish). Contrary to popular belief, rice, pasta, and potatoes are not bad for us, they are actually a great source of complex carbohydrates. It is what we put on them that can be fattening.

3. *Keep sugar and fat to a minimum.* Rather than count calories, count our grams of fat by reading package labels. Try to keep our daily fat intake to less than 30–40 grams. Use low fat or non fat dairy products, trim the fat off meat and chicken, choose tuna packed in water, and low fat salad dressings.

   Less dietary fat means less body fat, lower cholesterol levels and lower risk of colon cancer, breast cancer, and heart disease. Try to keep our sugar to a minimum by eating wholesome snacks (fruit, yogurt, pretzels, light ice cream).

   Stay away from products that contain saccharin, it has been known to cause cancer. Instead use real sugar in limited quantities.

4. *Drink coffee and caffeinated* sodas in moderation. Too much caffeine can increase our anxieties, interrupt our sleeping patterns, wreak havoc on our digestive system, and sometimes even cause our symptoms to intensify.

5. *Treat yourself right.* Don't deprive yourself of those occasional no-no's: french fries, ice cream, chicken-fried steak, gravy, butter, etc. When we deprive ourself of foods we enjoy we set ourself up for binging on that particular food and then feeling guilty and ashamed. We can let ourself off the hook for a day or two and

enjoy those foods we know are not good for us. Plan our indulgences. Again, moderation is the key.

6. *Shake the salt habit.* Our taste for salt is a habit, one that we can undo if we want to. Reducing our dependence on salt can actually enhance our enjoyment of foods. A high salt diet is closely correlated to high blood pressure, bloating and weight swings.

7. *Foods and psychiatric medications.* Many psychiatric medications, particularly the antipsychotics cause us to crave carbohydrates. We tend to gain large amounts of weight which then leads to decreased self-esteem, frustration, and further depression. If we are taking medications that we feel are contributing to a weight gain, talk to our doctor about alternatives or strategies that may lessen the impact of the drug on our physical health. Try to choose healthy carbohydrates (fruit, bagels without cream cheese, pretzels, spaghetti) during this period.

8. *Drink lots of water!* Good for us, plus it is especially important for those on psychiatric medications that cause dehydration as a side effect.

9. *Keep meat intake to a minimum.* Many of us grew up with the focus of our dinners being around a piece of meat every night. Over the years we've come to learn that excessive amounts of red meat can lead to high cholesterol levels, and high levels of triglycerides (fat) in the blood stream. Consequences include: increased risk of heart disease, stroke, obesity, breast and colon cancer. If you are a meat lover, try to eat it once or twice a week. Choose lean cuts (80% fat free or higher) and broil not fry. Not only will we save money, but we'll reduce the amount of fat in our diet and lose weight.

Suggestions for Good Food Choices

Breakfast
- Cereal with skim/low fat milk (Cheerios, Wheaties, Total, Raisin Bran, Oatmeal, Shredded Wheat)
- Bagels with low fat margarine/low fat cream cheese
- Bran muffins
- Fresh fruit
- Low fat/no fat yogurt
- Pancakes with fruit and a small amount of syrup

Lunch
- Tuna fish with low calorie mayonnaise
- Soups
- Salad with low calorie dressing
- Low fat/no fat yogurt

- Fresh fruit

- Cold pasta (leftovers)

- Bagel sandwiches

- Pita sandwiches filled with vegetables and low fat cheese

- Peanut butter and jelly on whole wheat bread

Dinner

- Chicken without the skin

- Make our own pizza using skim mozzarella, tomato sauce

- Pasta dishes (use tomato sauce or olive oil instead of butter)

- Baked potatoes or mashed potatoes made with skim milk

- Rice

- Frozen or fresh vegetables (stay away from canned if we can, too much salt)

- Lean cuts of meat/fish

- Tossed salad with low fat dressing

Healthy snacks

- Popcorn (lite versions usually have less fat)

- Pretzels

- Graham crackers

- Fresh fruit

- Fruit juice

- Frozen no fat/low fat yogurt

- Popsicles

Medical Self-Care and Disease Prevention

We can have a major impact on our health simply by taking the time to become better informed about health choices and behaviors. The best prescription for disease prevention is informed self-care. The research has shown that people with mental illness suffer an unusually high number of secondary illnesses such as heart disease, hypertension, lung cancer, and diabetes (Massaro, 1992). Many recipients of mental health services do not even have a primary care physician.

Choosing a primary care physician and establishing a relationship is of paramount importance. He or she will help us become familiar with our body and how it works, so that we can be better aware when something is amiss. He or she will help us learn different self-examination techniques.

Smoking nicotine products causes cancer. Many people begin smoking when they become involved in the mental health system. Most people want to stop, but it is very difficult to do on our own. Consulting with a doctor is helpful as there are several different supports, both physiological and psychological, available to help us quit if we choose to.

Safe Social Behaviors

Recovery means taking back responsibility for our life. It also involves responsible decision making about the use of drugs and alcohol in our life. Alcohol and street drugs negate the effects of prescribed medications in our body and can worsen symptoms.

Practicing safe sex is of paramount importance in this time when AIDS and sexually transmitted diseases are rampant. We are all vulnerable; no matter our race, religion, or sexual preference. Thus, taking control of our life involves making responsible decisions about our social lifestyle that contribute to our overall wellness. Only we know what is in our best interests; but other consumers, case managers, social workers, counselors, doctors, and community agencies are available for support around these decisions.

Recovery from mental illness is a very personal journey. But, it is about living a fulfilling life, a healthy and happy life, and a long life. Improving our wellness can be a critical support as we begin to redefine who we are and what we want out of life. Taking control of our fitness, nutrition, and health is empowering and beneficial for our body and our soul.

Examples from the self-help literature:

Exercise and physical activity strengthen my body and serve as an emotional safety valve.

Establishing good patterns of rest and sleep, exercise, diet, and self-discipline.

Minimizing consumption of foods which have proved harmful to me—sugar, coffee, coke, and other stimulants.

Losing weight helped me to feel better about myself.

I exercise at a community health center. Completing my workout bolsters my self-esteem. When I am not feeling well, exercise is an important part of my day.

If I am feeling "blah" and apathetic, I sleep, regardless of the time of day or night. Then, when I awaken, I write down my dreams. The sleep refreshes me, and the dreams direct my waking life.

I like to buy and prepare my own meals. This gives me a greater measure of control over what goes into me than would eating in restaurants. And it's cheaper, too.

Table 4.3—Proactive Health Behaviors

Practicing good nutrition: avoid sugar, salt, fats, caffeine, etc.

Eating three regular meals per day

Not using alcohol

Not using tobacco

Not using street drugs

Using seat belts and practicing safe driving habits

Getting sufficient sleep (seven to eight hours per night)

Taking a nap

Taking twenty minutes per day for regular relaxation and meditation

Focusing attention on the present

Exercising three times per week (aerobic, strength, endurance and stretching)

Maintaining recommended body weight

Controlling blood pressure and cholesterol level

Developing and maintaining satisfying personal relationships

Expressing feelings

Having an ongoing source of support

Making commitments

Owning a pet

Having hobbies such as woodworking, gardening, collecting, etc.

Increasing knowledge and skills through education

Maintaining a comforting and healthy environment

Developing interests in others and larger community

Being aware of a larger purpose or meaning to your life

Numerous studies have shown that the more we practice these behaviors, the better our day-to-day health will be.

Practice Exercise 4.12

1. Have you ever exercised for an extended period of time in your life? Please describe the activities and try to remember how you felt physically and emotionally during this time.

2. What are some easy, practical ways you could include physical activity in your life that wouldn't cause you financial stress or emotional stress.

Practice Exercise 4.13

*L*ist all the foods you ate yesterday in the first column, and then in the second column suggest healthier substitutions. For example, if you drank whole milk, you could substitute low fat milk.

Food Diary   **Healthier Options**

Responding to Practice Exercises 4.7 to 4.13

1. What are your own feelings and reactions to *Practice Exercises 4.7 to 4.13?*

2. Authors' comments on *Practice Exercises 4.7 to 4.13*:

   Life doesn't end with stress management. Managing our stresses is an important step toward releasing our personal capacity to create, to produce, to enjoy, and to contribute.

   Join or create a peer support group for emotional support, direct problem solving, and advocacy. The group process can help us to deal directly with sources of stress, both internal and external. The group process can help us to face the fear and the pain in our life rather than deny it or feel victimized by it. Regular meetings can assist us in debriefing experiences and looking for solutions.

   When you look closely at your day, you realize that you already have structure. You just haven't noticed.

   Our negative thoughts have their own history. It may not be necessary to know their history, but it is important to know that our negative thoughts have been learned by us. We can now unlearn them and learn more positive, and more accurate thoughts.

   We often have more personal permission for some feelings and less personal permission for other feelings. We can increase our personal permission for all of our feelings.

   Alcohol, drugs, smoking, overwork, hyperactivity, and certain foods can increase our feeling of stress. Also, these coping mechanisms (which may become addictions) can cause us to deny problems and ignore healthier solutions.

Personal Journal/Notes

CHAPTER **5** *Enhancing Personal Meaning*

Acknowledging Our Accomplishments

Awareness of Our Own Recovery Process

*C*hange involves loss, and loss involves recovery. The more change shakes the foundations of who we are, the more it breaks the connections we take for granted, the more it shatters our dreams and fantasies; the deeper and more profound the recovery process. Shock, denial, depression, anger, and acceptance are the recovery processes we experience. The recovery process is complex and not necessary linear. We move forward; we move backward. Yet, each phase has its own natural challenges and solutions that need to be worked through to move on to the next phases. There are few great leaps in this process. There is only the wrestling, the struggling, the failing and trying again (hopefully without self-blame), and the small successes. The outcomes of the recovery process are greater autonomy and a renewed sense of identity.

wow!

very discouraging

Examples from the self-help literature:

Learning more about myself, my limits, and weaknesses and strengths.

Not letting my symptoms build up. It is easier to interrupt them and get some relief when they are at lower levels.

Deciding to begin my life over again, to adopt a new healthier style of living. Through meditation and introspection I have probed for my life's purpose and developed short-term and long-term goals to serve that purpose.

Medication and therapy were not the only factors that made me feel well. I had to create a life that gave me the structure, support, and meaning I needed.

I learned that I could become my own therapist, that I have learned to help myself.

I had to change my priorities and take better care of myself.

I modified my attitudes, becoming more accepting and non-judgmental of others.

I make a deliberate effort to reduce noise and distractions as much as possible. They tend to confuse me.

I have made an extensive study of my illness and have found education invaluable in understanding my illness, coming to terms with it, and dealing with it.

I don't fight with myself over my vices, such as smoking. I have taken a serious look at the costs and benefits of my vices, and decided, once and for all, to take it or to leave it. Thus, I have saved the energy wasted on ambivalence.

Practice Exercise 5.1 **Self-Care**

1. Make a list of things that you enjoy doing. They may be things you enjoy doing alone or with others. Include some things you enjoyed when you were five to ten years old.

2. How can you include these things in your daily life?

Personal Enrichment | **Build a Fulfilling Life for Ourself**

*W*e are not doing ourself or others a favor by discounting ourself. It is important to have some challenges and exciting things to do that we enjoy naturally. Focusing on important tasks, directions, and people in our life can be an important source of energy and satisfaction. We cannot take good care of others if we are not taking good care of ourself. Many people find it hard to do things for themselves. Yet when we do not act in our own best interest, we are not modeling "how to make it" to others.

Examples from the self-help literature:

Finding meaningful work.

Setting reasonable and attainable goals.

Doing simple, non-taxing, emotionally fulfilling work that needs doing. This creates greater confidence and strength and may lead to a position of higher responsibility and greater financial rewards.

A paying job gives me something to look forward to each day, and a skill to learn and improve.

My work increases my self-image and self-confidence.

Give Ourself the Time to Make the Changes We Want and Need

If we have not been coping successfully or have been feeling especially stressed, it may require two to three years of personal effort to turn our life around. This may seem excessive, but we probably have spent many more years than that learning to be the way we are now. We must believe that we are worth the time and effort we invest in ourself—because we are. Change involves a decision, but it also involves learning new behaviors, much practice, and substantial support. Change that we *do not* chose personally is almost impossible. Change that we do chose is merely very difficult.

Examples from the self-help literature:

I give myself a lot of time to make decisions. I am very ambivalent and pressure to come to a quick decision can immobilize me.

Not pushing myself or allowing others to push me too fast.

Learning to make a move when it is helpful—to a new living situation to a new job.

I had to learn that I could not "wish" away the illness. I could not will it not to be so.

I was able to go to several therapists who were really helpful to me and supported me. The weekly meetings were a high point in my life.

Practice Exercise 5.2   **Personal Enrichment**

1. Make a list of things that would be enriching to you. They may be things you could do alone or with others.

2. How can you include these things in your daily life?

Develop a More Useful Philosophy of Life

*C*reate a philosophy that involves personal meanings that support our efforts, and that understands and forgives our limitations. This might involve spiritual as well as philosophical aspects. It may contain beliefs that enhance our own feeling of worth and our belief in the worth of others. Rethinking our personal philosophy can also increase our awareness of, and openness to, what is real. Our perceptions are often clouded by past and current attitudes and beliefs that may need to be challenged. What we perceive as real may actually be our opinion. The awareness that our perceptions are limited can be distressing, but it can also loosen our rigidity and open us up to develop new experiences and interactions. A helpful personal philosophy can also help us to meet life and its challenges with more flexibility. It can encourage us to look for options when something doesn't work instead of feeling stuck.

Examples from the self-help literature:

I have learned to accept myself as a highly creative person. Every creative person pays a price for non-conformity, seeking "new edges" to peer over. Being creative does not always bring comfort. The ups and downs of the roller coaster ride of creativity are normal. I had to learn that to choose creativity meant taking what the territory offered.

Only after I had accepted my illness as a long-term one could I really do something about improving my life.

Accepting that this is a process that takes time and many struggles.

Perfectionism is my enemy. I don't look for the perfect self, or for the perfect mate. Maturity means accepting flaws in myself and others.

Practice Exercise 5.3   **1.**   What has been the most meaningful experience in your life?

2.   What is the most courageous thing you ever did?

3.   What are the personal qualities you like most about yourself?

Acknowledge Our Own Wants

*W*ants are important to people. Knowing what we want, seeking what we want, getting what we want, and enjoying what we want helps us feel more in charge of our life. At times, simply meeting our needs may be all that we can handle. Soon we will begin to recognize that we do not need to limit ourself to what we need. Having and satisfying our wants adds a qualitative boost to our life.

Some people may actually have been told that they can only want what qualifies as a valid need. This is a very limiting position to take. It forces us to justify our wants (e.g., the reason I want the ice cream is because it is good for me). Another version of this position is that we are taught that we can only want what is possible, or what is reasonable. Again this requires us to justify our wants in terms of some standard or value outside of ourselves. A final version of this position is that we can only want what others approve.

Wanting need not be justified. Wanting need not be rational. Wanting is just there. It does not have to be limited by any pre-conditions. We can want anything, and we can't have everything we want. Wanting is a natural phenomenon that is often trained out of us by the people and environments we live with. We are trained to limit our wanting, inhibiting the natural flow of a very healthy and creative process. We can trust our judgement and our experience as a useful guide to ourselves. And our judgement will be honed and sharpened using it with a full range of wants. Rather than limiting our wants before we have explored the possibilities fully, we should return to our natural state of wanting.

Practice Exercise 5.4   **Wants**

1.   List as many of your personal wants as possible. Do not consider
     their reasonableness.

2.   Review your list. How can you begin to build some of your wants
     into your life?

Responding to Practice Exercises 5.1 to 5.4

1. What are you own feelings and reactions to *Practice Exercises 5.1 to 5.4?*

2. Authors' comments on *Practice Exercises 5.1 to 5.4:*

   Focusing on strengths builds a sense of empowerment.

   Self-care is important. We need to take good care of ourself in order to have the energy to take care of others. We need to keep our cup full.

   Taking care of ourself models important behaviors and attitudes to others.

   Activities that are enriching also help to reduce our stress and increase our self-esteem.

Personal Journal/Notes

Personal Journal/Notes

CHAPTER **6** *Building Personal Support*

Connecting

We are not alone in experiencing the effects of our life experiences. This is clearly evidenced in the growth of the self-help and advocacy movements among a wide variety of constituencies over the past decade. We are able to reach out for support and advocacy from others who have had similar life experiences. The learnings from those who have sought this type of support and advocacy can be especially valuable in coping with daily stresses, problem-solving potential solutions, and recommending specific reforms.

Feeling confident about connecting and finding ways to connect with others is often difficult. Yet, connections to valued activities and people are very important to the recovery process (Blanch et al., 1994, in press). It helps to let people know we like them and want their company. We know how good that feels to us. Also, it helps to let people know how you want them to react, especially when you have strong feelings. Let people know how you want them to act when you are angry, scared, sad or happy. Often we get frustrated because people do not give us the support we want. Often this happens because we have not told them how they can support us.

Being clear about what we want from others and what others want from us, can help to limit our tendency to "rescue." We rescue others because we assume we know what people want before they ask. Or we assume they are too dumb to know the answer and we must come up with it for them. Or we assume we know how to lead people's lives better than they do. Helping people to ask for what they want, or to clarify what they want in order to ask for it, helps them to take charge of their own lives. When we avoid rescuing, we are recognizing and encouraging the other person's ability to think and solve problems. We also avoid expending our energy needlessly, and are less likely to become stressed.

Examples from the self-help literature:

Learning new social skills.

Knowing when to closet myself and when to open my closet door.

I took weekend workshops to develop my self-esteem, and increase my assertiveness, learning new communication skills so I could say what I mean and mean what I say, rather than using old ways of manipulating others in the hope that some of my needs would be met.

Joined a 12-step program for adult children of dysfunctional parents.

I joined a self-help project, writing a manual for consumers, that gave me reason to get out of my apartment two or three mornings a week. It also brought me into contact with other consumers and some professionals. This made me feel I was back in society and had something to contribute.

I began to get to know, in a casual way, people in my neighborhood. The small talk, the "good mornings," and "hellos" provide a sense of belonging, and acceptance.

Attending religious services gave structure to my Sunday mornings.

I saw the community as a valuable resource, and I was creative in finding ways to interact with it.

If I become overwhelmed in a social situation, I may temporarily withdraw by going into another room, or even the bathroom.

I make it a habit to be polite and respectful to service people: bus-drivers, cashiers, etc. This helps my self-esteem and improves the quality of life for all.

I try not to push people, especially my family, any harder than they want to be pushed. I consider not what they can give me, but what I can contribute to their well-being.

Basic Communication Skills

There are a series of communication skills that are basic to all satisfying relationships. Learning how to improve our communication skills is critical in our recovery because it allows us to connect more fully to our support system. Good communication skills also make it easier for us to articulate our needs and wants in life in a manner that has positive outcomes for us.

Usually people learn a style of communicating by experience or observing others in relationships. Often we discover that the communication skills we have are ineffective, leaving us lacking in confidence and self-esteem in our own relationships.

The four essential skills involved in effective communication are *attending*, *listening*, *responding*, and *initiating*. These skills have been developed and researched by many people in the human services field. The skills presented in this workbook are based primarily on the work of Carkhuff (1983) and Anthony, Cohen, and Farkas (1990).

- *Attending:* This skill involves looking at people directly, facing them squarely, making eye contact, observing them.

- *Listening:* This skill includes ignoring internal distractions, listening to content, listening to meaning of what someone has said.

- *Responding:* This skill means acknowledging what we have heard, sharing our perspectives and self-disclosing.

- *Initiating:* This skill involves asking for what we want, planning what we need to do to get what we want and then taking the steps to achieve it.

Practice Exercise 6.1

Both of my sisters are pregnant and ~~they are~~ their due dates are 3 days apart. These babies may have the same birthday.

I hear you say...
What I hear you saying...
combine w/ p. 90

Listening: Listening well requires excellent concentration. In order to concentrate we must rid our mind of any distractions that might interfere with our listening. The following is an exercise to help improve listening skills.

Directions:

1. Write down a statement of (10-15) words about your life or some aspect of yourself.

2. A group leader will lead group through deep breathing/relaxation exercise to rid the mind of distractions. *(One type might include taking 4 or 5 deep breaths with eyes closed and exhaling slowly, releasing tensions and disruptive thoughts.)*

3. Each group member takes a turn reading their personal statement two times. Other group members then try to write down verbatim what they heard. People read back their statement and match its accuracy to the original.

Responding to Content: A good response to the content of what was said means paraphrasing the meaning without parroting all the details, and being as concise as possible.

1. *Example: "I'm so tired. I don't know what to do. I try to keep up with everything: work, home, classes. But each day seems so long, by noon I'm already too tired to cope."*

   Response: You're saying there is so much to do that you don't have the energy to do it all.

2. *Example: "Well, she's finally talking to me again. It's not the same, but at least we're talking. I still feel awful about the things she thinks I said about her. I would never do or say anything to hurt her. I think too much of her."*

   Response: You're saying that you are slowly getting the misunderstanding straightened out and you're talking to each other again.

Practice: Practice responding to the content. Paraphrase the original expression by using different words to express the same content.

1. *Example: "Thanks for all the help you've given me this semester. I was pretty mixed up when I got here, but now I really feel I've got it together. I'm passing all my courses for the first time."*

   Response:
   "You're saying that...

   ..

2. *Example: "I can't believe it, I blew it again! I just don't seem to be able to think before I open my big mouth. This job was going so smoothly until I got mad and told off my supervisor."*

   Response:
   "You're saying that...

   ..

Responding to Feelings

Responding to feelings involves having a vocabulary of feeling words that you can interchange with the feeling word expressed by the person you are listening to.

Below is a list of feeling words organized by category and intensity. You may add to the list.

	High	*Medium*	*Low*
Excited	delirious	animated	alive
	intoxicated	charged	great
	exhilarated	thrilled	stirred
Surprised	astonished	amazed	overcome
	staggered	awed	rocked
	stupefied	jolted	startled
Happy	ecstatic	exalted	great
	exuberant	fantastic	lively
	triumphant	tickled	super
Satisfied	delighted	charmed	agreeable
	enchanted	gratified	glad
	satiated	full	nice
Affectionate	cherish	adore	admire
	revere	esteem	regard
	treasure	prize	value
Calm	pacified	collected	bland
	sedated	mellow	quiet
	serene	restful	undisturbed

(continued)

Responding to Feelings *(continued)*

	High	*Medium*	*Low*
Distressed	agony crushed tormented	afflicted pained troubled	bad ill at ease upset
Frightened	frantic terrified petrified	aghast dread threatened	cautious hesitant shaky
Anxious	baffled perplexed tangled	blocked confounded stressed	careful muddled uncertain
Sad	despair devasted pitiful	awful gloomy sullen	down low unhappy
Angry	enraged infuriated livid	bristle fuming indignant	annoyed crabby sore
Ashamed	humiliated mortified sinful	chagrined criminal derelict	contrite regretful shame

Practice Exercise 6.2   **Responding to Feelings: Increasing Your Feeling Word Vocabulary**

Directions: Take each of the stimulus words given and complete the sentence with another feeling word. Use the new word as your next stimulus and repeat the process.

Round Robin activity?

Example
When I feel *angry*, I feel *furious*,
When I feel *furious*, I feel *burned*,
When I feel *burned*, I feel *cheated*,
When I feel *cheated*, I feel *hurt*,
When I feel *hurt*, I feel *sad*.

Practice 1

When I feel *happy*, I feel ....,

When I feel ...., I feel ....,

When I feel ...., I feel ....,

When I feel ...., I feel ....,

When I fee ...., I feel ....

Practice 2

When I feel *overwhelmed*, I feel..,

When I feel ...., I feel ....,

When I feel ...., I feel ....,

When I feel ...., I feel ....,

When I feel ...., I feel ....

Practice 3

When I feel *afraid*, I feel ....,

When I feel ...., I feel ....,

When I feel ...., I feel ....,

When I feel ...., I feel ....,

When I feel ...., I feel ....

Practice Exercise 6.3   **Responding to Feelings: Empathy**

Directions: This exercise will help you learn to listen to other people's feelings and respond to them. Imagine you are listening to the people below. Try to respond to the feelings expressed. Use your feeling word chart. A helpful hint when listening empathetically is to ask yourself, "How would I feel if I were this person?" not "How would I feel in that situation?"

Example: *"Things are all straightened out with my daughter now. I explained to her about my drinking problem and why I have to go to these long meetings. It's still hard for her 'cause she's so young, but she understands a little better what Mommy does."*

Response: You feel *relieved.*
You feel *hopeful.*

Practice

1. *"Well, here I am again. It's mid-semester and I'm way behind in all my work, just barely passing a couple of courses. It's like I can't think ahead. I do the same thing every semester. What's wrong with me—can't I learn from my past?"*

Response: You feel...

You feel...

2. *"I'm just a three quartersman. I've had so many opportunities in my life and I've thrown them all away."*

Response: You feel...

You feel...

3. *"I'm really excited about this new job. I'm starting out at the bottom and the work is pretty dull right now, but there's so much to learn! The potential for advancement is really good."*

Response: You feel...

You feel...

[handwritten notes in left margin:] You shouldn't tell someone how they are feeling! Acknowledge & Ask questions back — combine w/ page 86

Initiating

Initiating means acting to change or improve a personal experience. Learning how to initiate is a crucial skill in our recovery because it allows us to take action in the areas of our life that we want to improve or change. (Initiating will be covered in detail in Chapter Seven.)

Save for Ch 7

Initiating involves

1. *Operationalizing our goal:* writing our goal so that it is observable and measurable.

2. *Initiating steps to the goal:* Figuring out the steps it will take to reach the goal.

3. *Developing a schedule for completing the steps:* Writing a plan or program that sequences the steps we need to take to reach our goal.

4. *Reinforcing ourself for the achievement of our goals:* Planning rewards for each step we achieve as a way to motivate ourself to pursue our goals.

Example

Personalized problem

I feel frustrated because I don't know how to go about looking for a job and I want to learn how.

Goal

I will attend the Career Education Program three times/week to develop a career plan.

Steps

1. Call Career Education Program for information. *(reinforcer: buy a new tape)*

2. Fill out application to Career Education Program. *(reinforcer: have coffee with a friend)*

3. Attend interview for Career Education Program. *(reinforcer: buy new earrings)*

4. Attend classes. *(reinforcer: buy a new sweater)*

Asking for Support

Steps in Seeking Support

1. Be clear with yourself about what you want (listening, advice, stroking, feedback, etc.)

2. Be clear with the other person about what you want from him/her.

3. Ask whether he/she is willing to give it to you.

4. If he/she is not willing to give it to you now, ask when will he/she be willing?

5. If he/she is not willing to give it to you at all, what is he/she willing to do or give.

6. If you cannot get the support you need from him/her, try someone else.

Practice Exercise 6.4 **Building Social Support**

1. Name three people you do or can use for support/activities.

2. How do you like to be supported when you are angry? What do you want people around you to do? Be specific.

3. How do you like to be supported when you are scared? What do you want people around you to do? Be specific.

4. How do you like to be supported when you are sad? What do you want people around you to do. Be specific.

5. How do you like to be supported when you are happy? What do you want people around you to do? Be specific.

Practice Exercise 6.5 **Getting Personal Support**

1. Think of an issue around which you want some support.
    Write the issue down.

2. What kind of support do you want around this issue?
    Be as specific as possible?

3. Who do you want this support from?

4. What do you want from this person? Be as specific as possible.

Setting Boundaries on Our Relationships

The process of learning to set boundaries on our relationships is difficult. One example of setting boundaries is learning to manage situations we cannot or need not assume responsibility for. The judgement involved in deciding what to respond to and how to respond can be influenced by our family, friends, and knowledgeable professionals. The benefit of learning to set boundaries is the possibility of refocusing our energy in more useful directions. We will be surprised at what we can walk away from. The ability to set boundaries allows us to gain a new perspective and a new resolve to engage our life in more valued ways.

Sometimes we find ourself rescuing others when we really don't want to. Rescuing is a very draining activity. Rescuing means:

- Doing something for others that they can reasonably do for themselves.

- Assuming we know what the other person wants or needs.

- Not doing something because of its assumed effect, such as not saying something because we assume the other person cannot handle it.

- Doing something for someone that we really don't want to do.

Rescuing is a way of helping others that really discounts them and ourself. It denies our own boundaries, our feelings and wants, and it does not acknowledge what the other person wants. Rescuing frequently leaves us feeling hurt because our helping does not really meet the need of the person. We then become angry at the person we have rescued because they are not grateful. It can be a dangerous triangle.

How to Help Without Rescuing

1. Ask the person what he/she wants and doesn't want.

2. Be clear about what we want to do and what we don't want to do.

3. Be clear about what we are capable of and what we are not capable of.

4. Negotiate with the other person what we will and what we will not do.

5. Acknowledge that we may have an investment in rescuing others—and find out why.

Practice Exercise 6.6   **1.**   Describe a situation in which you tend to rescue another person.

2.   What would you like to do differently? Be clear about what you want or don't want to do.

3.   What is most likely to go wrong? How can you deal with this?

4.   What is most likely to go right?

Responding to Practice Exercises 6.1 to 6.6

1. What are your own feelings and reactions to *Practice Exercises 6.1 to 6.6?*

2. Authors' comments on *Practice Exercises 6.1 to 6.6:*

    People with mental illness do not have a "problem." They have a disability. Negative personal and societal attitudes and beliefs create the "problem."

    We often assume what people want when they have strong feelings (e.g., anger, scare, sadness, happiness). We assume people want what we want. This may not be accurate. It is more helpful to ask people what they want.

Personal Journal/Notes

CHAPTER 7 *Setting Personal Goals*

A Step-by-Step Guide for Setting Personal Goals

The previous chapters have given us an opportunity to assess our symptoms and sources of stress. We have been able to explore the content of our stress and some of the sources that give rise to our symptoms. This chapter will help us to further personalize several key stress issues/problems, to understand their meaning to us, to identify behaviors that prevent us from dealing effectively with the issues/problems, and to help us to translate the issues/problems into personal stress management goals. In effect, we will be given a process that is independent of the specific content of our issues/problems. This process will make us a better problem solver. This process is based on the work of Carkhuff (1983) and Anthony, Cohen, and Farkas (1990).

A further clarification of the concept "issue/problem" may be useful to the reader. It is helpful to view stress related issues/problems, whether their source is internal or external to us; as information, skill, or support deficits. Having issues or problems is often interpreted as having something wrong with us. This can leave us feeling badly or discounted. More important, this approach does not provide any direction or even hope for solutions to the issues or problems. Viewing our issues/problems as knowledge, skill or support deficits removes the image of "badness or wrongness" and provides a concrete direction for what to do. If we are unable or unwilling to do something it is because we lack the knowledge, skills or supports to be effective. We can learn the necessary knowledge and skills and we can get more useful support to deal effectively with our sources of stress. This developmental perspective removes blaming and helps people to become more knowledgeable, skillful, and better supported.

Practice Exercise 7.1

1. What are some of the major stress issues/problems that you identified in the previous chapters?

   Examples: *Stigma*
   Too many demands on my time

   a.

   b.

   c.

   d.

   e.

   f.

   g.

   h.

2. Share your responses with the group.

Practice Exercise 7.2

1. Choose one stress management issue/problem from *Practice Exercise 7.1* that you want to work on during the remaining sessions. Your choice may be based upon the urgency of the issue/problem, how easily you can resolve it, or your level of motivation to resolve it. Restate the stress management issue/problem in terms of how it affects you. What is its impact on you? Identify a key feeling/symptom associated with it.

   Example: *I feel angry because I am worn out by the demands people make on me.*

   I feel...because I...
   ....
   ....
   ....

2. Develop and share your responses with the group.

Practice Exercise 7.3

1. Restate the issue/problem statement in *Practice Exercise 7.2* in terms of something you are not doing or cannot do. Describe specific behaviors.

Example: I feel angry because I am not setting limits on, or saying no to, the demands people make on me.

I feel...because I can not (am not) ....

....

....

....

2. Develop and share your responses with the group.

Practice Exercise 7.4   **1.**   Restate the issue/problem statement in *Practice Exercise 7.3* in terms of a goal for yourself. The goal should be the opposite of what you cannot do or are not doing. Be as specific and as behavioral as possible. Do not introduce any new behavior not mentioned in *Practice Exercise 7.3*.

Example: I want to set limits on or say no to the demands people make on me.

Goal: I want..

....

....

....

2.   Develop and share your responses with the group.

Practice Exercise 7.5

1. Identify the information, skills, or support required to reach your stress management goal statement. Do not be concerned at this point about whether you have the information, skills, or support. Simply list what is needed.

Example: Support from my friends; learning how to say no; setting priorities on what I want to do; acknowledging that I do not have to solve everyone's problems; accepting my own limitations.

Goal: *Needed information/skills/support*

Information

Skills

Support

2. Develop and share your responses with the group.

Developing a Plan for a Personal Goal

The purpose of this section is to help us develop a systematic plan for achieving a personal goal. This section may be too detailed and specific for some people. Also, certain more easily identified and achievable stress management goals may not require this level of planning. However, in the authors' opinion, the point at which the change process is most vulnerable is in the implementation and maintenance phases. This is where the lack of knowledge, skills, or support begins to show up. And without adequate knowledge, skills, and support our best laid plans may not work out. A well thought-out plan increases the likelihood that our goals will be achieved, and that we will weather the inevitable frustrations and failures that accompany any significant change process. A good plan does not necessarily make the change process any easier, but it may make it more likely.

Developing a plan for a personal goal includes: identifying steps/activities required to reach the goal; sequencing the steps/activities; setting time lines for each step; identifying the person responsible for carrying out each step; developing a format for monitoring the achievement of each step; and identifying resources for achieving the goals and steps/activities.

Practice Exercise 7.6

1. In this exercise you will be listing the steps/activities necessary to accomplish your goal. You will be using your goal statement in *Practice Exercise 7.4* and the information in *Practice Exercise 7.5* in developing the steps/activities.

   Example Goal Statement: *I want to set limits on, or say no to, the demands people make on me.*

Steps/Activities	Potential Resources
_4_ Practice saying no to people in general.	Friends
_3_ Talk about my decision to set better limits; to validate my own needs and wants; to accept my own strengths and limitations.	Friend Therapist
_2_ Talk about my need to rescue other people.	Friend Therapist
_1_ Spend time thinking about what I want to do; what are my priorities.	Myself Friend
_5_ Keep a record of how I actually set better limits on my time; when I say no.	Myself

2. Write down goal statement from *Practice Exercise 7.4.*

3. List the steps/activities needed to reach your goal statement. Use the information from *Practice Exercise 7.5* to develop the steps/activities. List as many as possible. Do not be concerned about their order at this time. Develop and share your responses with your partner.

Steps/Activities   *Potential Resources*

___ **a.**

___ **b.**

___ **c.**

___ **d.**

___ **e.**

___ **f.**

4. Put the steps/activities in the order you want to accomplish them by placing the appropriate number in front of each step/activity.

5. For each step/activity, identify potential resources for accomplishing it.

6. Write the goal statement and steps/activities in the form on the following page.

7. Identify the person responsible for each step/activity.

8. Identify expected dates of completion for each step/activity.

Practice Exercise 7.6
continued

Personal Goal Plan and Monitoring Form

Goal Statement:

Beginning Date:

Steps/ Activities	Person Responsible	Expected Date of Completion

9. Develop and discuss your responses with the group.

Practice Exercise 7.7

1. What are some things you learned about yourself as a result of this chapter and discussion?

a.

b.

c.

2. Share your responses with the group.

Responding to Practice Exercises 7.1 to 7.7

1. What are your own feelings and reactions to *Practice Exercises 7.1 to 7.7?*

2. Authors' comments on *Practice Exercises 7.1 to 7.7:*

    People with mental illness do not have a "problem." They have a disability. Negative personal and societal attitudes and beliefs create the "problem."

    We often assume what people want when they have strong feelings (e.g., anger, scare, sadness, happiness). We assume people want what we want. This may not be accurate. It is more helpful to ask people what they want.

Personal Journal/Notes

Personal Journal/Notes

Bibliography

Anonymous. (1980). After the funny farm. *Schizophrenia Bulletin, 6(3),* 544–546.

Anonymous. (1981). The quiet discrimination. *Schizophrenia Bulletin, 7(4),* 736–738.

Anonymous. (1983). Schizophrenia—A pharmacy student's view. *Schizophrenia Bulletin, 9(1),* 152–155.

Anonymous. (1983). A father's thoughts. *Schizophrenia Bulletin, 9(3),* 439–442.

Anonymous. (1989). How I've managed chronic mental illness. *Schizophrenia Bulletin, 15(4),* 635–640.

Anonymous. (1990). A pit of confusion. *Schizophrenia Bulletin, 16(2),* 355–359.

Anonymous. (1990). Behind the mask: A functional schizophrenic copes. *Schizophrenia Bulletin 16(3),* 547–549.

Anthony, W.A. (1993). Recovery from mental illness: The guiding vision of the mental health service system in the 1990s. *Psychosocial Rehabilitation Journal, 16(4),* 11–23.

Anthony, W.A., Cohen, M.R., & Farkas, M.D. (1990). *Psychiatric Rehabilitation.* Boston: Boston University, Center for Psychiatric Rehabilitation.

Augoustinos, M. (1986). Psychiatric inpatients' attitudes toward mental disorder and the tendency to adopt a sick-role. *Psychological Reports, 58,* 495–498.

Bellingham, R., Cohen, B., Jones, T. & Spaniol, L. (1989). Connectedness: Some skills for spiritual health. *American Journal of Health Promotion,* 18–24 & 31.

Biegel, D.E., Sales, E., & Schulz, R. (1991). *Family caregiving in chronic illness.* Newbury Park, CA: Sage Publishers.

Blanch, A., Fisher, D., Tucker, W., Walsh, D. & Chassman, J. (1994, in press). Consumer-practitioners and psychiatrists share insights about recovery and coping. *Disability Studies Quarterly.*

Boffey, P.M., Eckholm, E., Schmeck, H.M. & Goleman, D. (1986). Schizophrenia: A series that looks at the problems, the toll, the strains on families—and the hopes for the future. New York: *The New York Times*, March 16, 17, 18, & 19. (Available in booklet form from NAMI).

Bond, G.R. & De Graaf-Kaser, R. (1990). Group approaches for persons with severe mental illness: A typology. In *Group work with the emotionally disabled*. Haworth Press, Inc.

Borck, L.E., Aber, R.A. (1981). The enhancing of social support for mental health patients through the development of self-help groups. *Community Support Services Journal, 2,* 11–15.

Borkman, T. (1984). Mutual self-help groups: Strengthening the selectively unsupportive personal and community networks of their members. In A. Gartner & F. Reissman (Eds.), *The self-help revolution*. New York: Human Services Press, 205–216.

Breier, A. & Strauss, J.S. (1983). Self-control in psychotic disorders. *Archives of General Psychiatry, 40,* 1141–1145.

Breier, A. & Strauss, J.S. (1984). The role of social relationships in the recovery from psychotic disorders. *American Journal of Psychiatry, 141(8),* 949–955.

Brodoff, A.S. (1988). Schizophrenia through a sister's eyes—the burden of invisible baggage. *Schizophrenia Bulletin, 14(1),* 113–116.

Brundage, B. (1983). What I wanted to know but was afraid to ask. *Schizophrenia Bulletin, 9(4),* 583–585.

Burton, A., Lopez-Ibor, J.J. & Mendel, W.M. (1974). *Schizophrenia as a lifestyle*. New York: Springer Publishing Co.

Caldwell-Smith, G. (1990). A mother's view. *Schizophrenia Bulletin, 16(4).*

Carkhuff, R.R. (1983). *The art of helping, 5th edition*. Amherst, MA: Human Resource Development Press.

Center for Psychiatric Rehabilitation. (1988). Consumer/ex-patient initiatives. *Community Support Network News, 5(2).*

Chamberlin, J. (1978). *On our own: Patient controlled alternatives to the mental health system*. New York: McGraw Hill.

Chamberlin, J. (1984). Speaking for ourselves: An overview of the ex-psychiatric inmates' movement. *Psychosocial Rehabilitation Journal, 8(2),* 56–63.

Chamberlin, J. (1990). The ex-patients movement: Where we've been and where we're going. *The Journal of Mind and Behavior, 11(3&4),* 323–336.

Cohen, C.I. & Berk, L.A. (1985). Personal coping styles of schizophrenic outpatients. *Hospital and Community Psychiatry, 36(4),* 407–410.

Cohen, M.B., Nemec, P.B., Farkas, M.D., & Forbes, R. (1988). *Psychiatric rehabilitation training technology: Case management*. Boston: Boston University, Center for Psychiatric Rehabilitation.

Consumer First-Person Narratives. (1991). *Psychosocial Rehabilitation Journal,15(2)*, 7–18.

Copeland, M.E. (1991). *Learning to cope with depression and manic depression.* Brattleboro, Vt.: Peach Press.

Davidson, L. & Strauss, J.S. (1992). Sense of self in recovery from severe mental illness. *British Journal of Medical Psychology, 65*, 131–145.

Davis, M., Robbins Eshelman, E. and McKay, M. (1991) *The relaxation and stress reduction workbook, Third edition.* Oakland, CA: New Harbinger Publications.

Deegan, P. (1988). Recovery: The lived experience of rehabilitation. *Psychosocial Rehabilitation Journal, 11(4)*, 11–19.

Deegan, P. (1992). The independent living movement and people with psychiatric disabilities: Taking control back over our own lives. *Psychosocial Rehabilitation Journal, 15(3)*, 3–20.

Duval, M. (1979). Giving love ... and schizophrenia. *Schizophrenia Bulletin, 5(4)*, 631–636.

Easwaran, E. (1978). *Meditation: An eight point program.* Nilgiri Press.

Edmundson, E. et al. (1982). Integrating skill building and peer support in mental health treatment. In A. Yaeger & R. Slotnik (Eds.), *Community Mental Health and Behavioral Ecology* (pp. 127–139). New York: Plenum.

Emerick, R.E. (1990). Self-help groups for former patients; Relations with mental health professionals. *Hospital and Community Psychiatry, 41(4)*, 401–407.

Estroff, S.E. (1981). *Making it crazy: An ethnography of psychiatric clients in an American community.* Berkeley: University of California Press.

Fortner, R. (1988). The history and outcome of my encounter with schizophrenia. *Schizophrenia Bulletin, 14(4)*, 701–706.

Fuchs, L. (1986). Three generations of schizophrenia. *Schizophrenia Bulletin, 12(4)*, 744–747.

Gartner, A.J. & Riessman, F. (1982). Self-help and mental health. *Hospital and Community Psychiatry, 33(8)*, 631–635.

Goffman, E. (1961). Asylums: *Essays on the social situation of mental patients and other inmates.* Garden City. M.Y.: Anchor Books, Doubleday and Company.

Grof, S. (1988). *The adventure of self-discovery: Dimensions of consciousness and new perspectives in psychotherapy and inner exploration.* Albany: State University of New York Press.

Harding, C.M., Zubin, J. & Strauss, J.S. (1992). Chronicity in schizophrenia: Revisited. *British Journal of Psychiatry, 161(suppl. 18)*, 27–37.

Harp, H. (1987). Philosophical models. In S. Zinman, H.T. Harp, & S. Bud (Eds.). *Reaching across: Mental health clients helping each other* (pp. 19–24). Riverside, CA: California Network of Mental Health Clients.

Houghton, J. F. (1982). Maintaining mental health in a turbulent world. *Schizophrenia Bulletin, 8(3)*, 548–552.

Houston, J. (1992). Myths of the future. *Humanistic Psychologist, 20(1)*, 4–17.

Jacobs, M. & Goodman, G. (1989). Psychology and self-help groups. *American Psychologist, 3*, 536–545.

Jurik, N. (1987). Persuasion in a self-help group: Processes and consequences. *Small Group Behavior*, August.

Kanter, J. (1985). The process of change in the long-term mentally ill: A naturalistic perspective. *Psychosocial Rehabilitation Journal, 9(1)*, 55–69.

Kelly, D.M., Sautter, F., Tugrul, K. & Weaver, M.D. (1990). Fostering self-help on an inpatient unit. *Archives of Psychiatric Nursing, IV(3)*, 161–165.

Kiev, A. (Ed.) (1964). *Magic, faith, and healing: Studies in primitive psychiatry today*. New York: Free Press of Glencoe.

Kivnick, H.Q. and Erikson J.M. (1983). The arts as healing. *American Journal of Orthopsychiatry, 53(4)*, 602–617.

Knight, B., Wollert, R., Levy, L.H., Frame, C.L., & Padgett, V. (1980). Self-help groups: The members' perspectives. *American Journal of Community Psychology, 8*, 53–64.

Kurtz, L.F. & Powell, T.J. (1987). Three approaches to understanding self-help groups. *Social Work with Groups, 10(3)*, 69–80.

Lazarus, R.S. (1976). *Patterns for adjustment*. New York: McGraw-Hill.

Lazarus, R.S. & Folkman, S. (1984). *Stress, appraisal, and coping*. New York: Springer.

Leavy, R.L. (1983). Social support and psychological disorder: A review. *Journal of Community Psychology, 11*, 3–21.

Leete, E. (1987). The treatment of schizophrenia: A patient's perspective. *Hospital and Community Psychiatry, 38(5)*, 486–491.

Leete, E. (1988). The role of the consumer movement and persons with mental illness. *1988 Switzer Monograph*. National Rehabilitation Association.

Leete, E. (1988). A consumer perspective on psychosocial treatment. *Psychosocial Rehabilitation Journal, 12(2)*, 45–52.

Leete, E. (1989). How I perceive and manage my illness. *Schizophrenia Bulletin, 15(2)*, 197–200.

Levy, L. (1981). The national schizophrenia fellowship: A British self-help group. *Social Psychiatry, 16*, 129–135.

Massaro, R.P. (1992). The impact of physical health problems on psychiatric rehabilitation technology. *Psychosocial Rehabilitation Journal, 15(3)*, 113–118.

McDermott, B. (1990). Transforming depression. *The Journal of CAMI, 1(4),* 13–14.

McGrath, M.E. (1984). Where did I go? *Schizophrenia Bulletin, 10(4),* 638–690.

Minor, D. (1981). Third side of the coin. *Schizophrenia Bulletin, 7(2),* 316–317.

National Association of State Mental Health Program Directors. (1989). Position paper on consumer contributions to mental health service delivery systems endorsed by membership.

National Institute of Mental Health. (undated). *You are not alone: facts about mental health and mental illness.* Rockville, MD: National Institute of Mental Health.

Nicholaichuk, T.P. & Wollert, R. (1989). The effects of self-help on health status and health-services utilization. *Canadian Journal of Community Mental Health, 8,* 17–29.

Nichols, D.A. (1988). A critique of shelter living. *Psychosocial Rehabilitation Journal, 12(1),* 66–68.

O'Neal, J.M. (1984). Finding myself and loving it. *Schizophrenia Bulletin, 10(1),* 109–110.

Paulson, R.I. (1991). Professional training for consumers and family members: One road to empowerment. *Psychosocial Rehabilitation Journal, 14(3),* 69–80.

Piercey, B.P. (1985). First person account: Making the best of it. *Schizophrenia Bulletin, 11(1),* 156–157.

Powell, T. (1987). *Self-help groups and professional practice.* Washington, D.C.: National Association of Social Workers.

Rappaport, J. (1981). In praise of paradox: A social policy of empowerment over prevention. *American Journal of Community Psychology, 9(1),* 1–5.

Rappaport, J. (1985). The power of empowerment language. *Social Policy, 16(2),* 15–20.

Research and Training Center on Community Living (1990). *Effective self-advocacy: Empowering people with disabilities to speak for themselves.* Minneapolis Institute on Community Living.

Rogers, J.A. & Centifanti, J.B. (1988). Madness, myths, and reality: Response to Roberta Rose. *Schizophrenia Bulletin, 14(1),* 7–14.

Ruocchio, P.J. (1991). The schizophrenic inside. *Schizophrenia Bulletin, 17(2),* 357–360.

Segal, S.P., Silverman, C. & Temkin, T. (1991). Enabling, empowerment, and self-help agency practice. *Workshop on Consumer-Led Self-Help Services,* NIMH, Rockville, MD, March 6.

Selye, H. (1974). *Stress without distress.* Philadelphia: Lippincott.

Shaffer, M. (1982). *Life after stress.* New York: Plenum Press.
Sherman, P.S. & Porter, R. (1991). Mental health consumers as case management aides. *Hospital and Community Psychiatry, 42(5),* 494–498.

Silverman, C., Segal, S., & Anello, E. (1989). Community and the homeless and mentally disabled: The structure of self-help groups. (Paper presented at 1987 American Psychological Association Annual Meeting in San Francisco). Berkeley, CA.

Simon, B. (1990). Rethinking empowerment. *Journal of Progressive Human Services, 1(1)*, 27–37.

Skrinar, G.S., Hutchinson, D.S., & Williams, N. (1992). Exercise: An adjunct therapy for persons with psychiatric disabilities. *Medical Science, Sports, and Exercise, 24(5)*, 536, supplement.

Smith, R.T. (1979). Disability and the recovery process: Role of social networks. In E.G. Jaco (Ed.). *Patients, physicians and illness* (pp. 218–226). New York: The Free Press.

Spaniol, L. (1993). *Beyond stress management: A holistic approach.* Boston: Boston University, Center for Psychiatric Rehabilitation.

Spaniol, L. & Lannan, P. (1984). *Getting unstuck: Moving on after divorce.* New York: Paulist Press.

Spaniol, L. & Koehler, M. (1993). *The experience of recovery.* Boston: Boston University, Center for Psychiatric Rehabilitation.

Strauss, J.S. (1986). Discussion: What does rehabilitation accomplish? *Schizophrenia Bulletin, 12(4)*, 720–723.

Strauss, J.S. (1992). The person—key to understanding mental illness: Towards a new dynamic psychiatry, III. *British Journal of Psychiatry, 161(suppl. 18)*, 19–26.

Strauss, J.S., Hafez, H., Liberman, P. & Harding, C.M. (1985). The course of psychiatric disorder, III: Longitudinal principles. *American Journal of Psychiatry, 142(3)*, 289–296.

Szasz, T.S. (1970). *The manufacture of madness.* New York: Harper Colothon Books, Harper and Row.

Thompson, E.H. (1989). Recovery networks and patient interpretations of mental illness. *Journal of Community Psychology, 17*, 5–15.

Torrey, E.F. (1988). *Surviving schizophrenia: A family manual. Revised Edition.* New New York: Harper and Row.

Unzicker, R. (1989). On my own: A personal journey through madness and re-emergence. *Psychosocial Rehabilitation Journal, 13(1)*, 71–77.

Van Den Bosch, R.J., Van Asma, M.J.O., Rombouts, R. & Louwerens, J.W. (1992). Coping style and cognitive dysfunction in schizophrenic patients. *British Journal of Psychiatry, 161(suppl. 18)*, 123–128.

Wexler, D., Colborn, J., & Jacobus, R. (1992). *A consumers guide to cooperative housing.* Champlain Valley Mutual Housing Federation, c/o BCLT, PO Box 523, Burlington, VT 05402, 802-862-5430.

Wiedl, K.H. (1992). Assessment of coping with schizophrenia: Stressors, appraisals, and coping behavior. *British Journal of Psychiatry, 161(suppl. 18)*, 114–122.

Wiedl, K.H. & Schottner, B. (1991). Coping with symptoms related to schizophrenia. *Schizophrenia Bulletin, 17(3),* 525–538.

Wilson, H.S. (1984). The rotten apple stigma: Diagnostic labeling. *Journal of Psychosocial Nursing and Mental Health Services.* October.

Wollert, R. (1986). Psychosocial helping processes in a heterogeneous sample of self-help groups. *Canadian Journal of Mental Health, 5,* 63–76.

Woodman, T. (1987). A pessimist's progress. *Schizophrenia Bulletin, 13(2),* 329–331.

Young, J. & Williams, C.L. (1988). Whom do mutual-help groups help? A typology of members. *Hospital and Community Psychiatry, 39(11),* 1178–1182.

Zellerbach Family Fund. (1989). *Clients serving clients.* San Francisco Study Center, San Francisco, California.

Zinman, S. (1982). A patient-run residence. *Psychosocial Rehabilitation Journal, 6(1),* 3–11.

Zinman, S. (1986). Self-help: The wave of the future. *Hospital and Community Psychiatry, 37(3),* 213.

Zinman, S. (1987). Definition of self-help groups. In S. Zinman, H.T. Harp, & S. Bud (Eds.). *Reaching across: Mental health clients helping each other* (pp. 19–24). Riverside, CA: California Network of Mental Health Clients.

Zubin, J., Steinhauer, S.R. & Condray, R. (1992). Vulnerability to relapse in schizophrenia. *British Journal of Psychiatry, 161(suppl. 18),* 13–18.